PEDIATRICS - LABORATORY AND CLINICAL RESEARCH

THE OPTIMIZATION OF DRUG PRESCRIBING IN CHILDREN

PEDIATRICS - LABORATORY AND CLINICAL RESEARCH

Additional books in this series can be found on Nova's website under the Series tab.

Additional e-books in this series can be found on Nova's website under the eBooks tab.

PEDIATRICS - LABORATORY AND CLINICAL RESEARCH

THE OPTIMIZATION OF DRUG PRESCRIBING IN CHILDREN

HUGO JUAREZ OLGUIN
EDITOR

nova
biomedical
New York

Library of Congress Cataloging-in-Publication Data

ISBN: 978-1-53612-263-3

Published by Nova Science Publishers, Inc. † New York

Contents

Preface vii

Acknowledgments xiii

Chapter 1 Pharmacokinetics and Its Clinical Applications **1**
Ismael Lares-Asseff and Hugo Juarez Olguín

Chapter 2 Pharmacokinetic, Growth and Development **25**
Ismael Lares-Asseff and Gabriela Pérez Guille

Chapter 3 Main Diseases in Pediatrics **51**
Mayra Santillán García, Monica Punzo Soto and Belen Juarez Tapia

Chapter 4 How Is the LADME Process of Drugs in Children? **75**
Hugo Juarez Olguín, David Calderón Guzmán and Mónica Punzo Soto

Chapter 5 Pharmacology for the Fetus and the Newborn **91**
Hugo Juarez Olguín and Ismael Lares-Asseff

Chapter 6	Pharmacokinetic Principles in the Use of Antibiotics in Pediatrics *María-Gabriela Pérez Guille, Ismael Lares-Asseff and Alejandra Toledo López*	**113**
Chapter 7	Therapeutic Drug Monitoring in Children *Hugo Juarez Olguín, Monica Punzo Soto and Belen Juárez Tapia*	**133**
Chapter 8	Nutrition and Pharmacokinetics of Medicines *Ismael Lares-Asseff, Mayra Santillán García and Belen Juarez Tapia*	**155**
Chapter 9	Pharmacovigilance and Pharmacoepidemiology of Drugs in a Pediatric Hospital *Hugo Juarez Olguín, Fernanda Reyes Gonzalez and Janett Flores Perez*	**189**
Chapter 10	Unintentional Drug Poisoning in the Pediatric Population *Hugo Juarez Olguín, Carmen Flores Pérez and Janett Flores Pérez*	**203**
Chapter 11	Suicidal Attempts by Consumption of Drugs in Children *Mónica Punzo Soto, Carmen Flores Pérez and Mayra Santillán García*	**213**
Index		**221**

PREFACE

Pediatrics is the form of medical care that is concerned with children from birth to adolescence, specializing in a variety of characteristics and changes subjective to each patient. Undoubtedly, these changes influence drug distribution and response. The body composition and the processes of biological and physiological maturation constitute important variables worthy of consideration in the effort to adequately satisfy the therapeutic necessities of all the age groups, since different formulations are required to achieve optimum therapy.

The technological advances in the last decades have endowed humanity with the facilities to painstakingly analyze biological samples and thus give way to potential progress in pharmacokinetics and pharmacodynamics. From this knowledge, it becomes clear that the body is a dynamic model and thus, brings to light the necessity to individualize treatment regimens based on parameters of each and every individual, which in the past was not as important.

There are instruments that contribute to optimizing drug management and safety in the pediatric population as recommended by the World Health Organization that rotate on the application of drug monitoring strategies that would contribute to ensuring the safety of patients and improve treatment schemes with increasingly safe and effective drugs. Furthermore, recourses to the therapeutic monitoring of drugs would become available where a monitoring based principally on the drug plasma levels is carried out in order to make the pertinent dose adjustments. The need for this will arise, since the most effective therapeutic range of many drugs is still unknown; unnecessarily high concentrations with potential risks of producing toxicity in patients is something that must be avoided. With these factors in mind, the decision to compose this book for pediatric doctors as well as specialists in the health sector who are dedicated to childcare became apparent, with the hope of portraying an array of pharmacokinetic knowledge, based on new therapeutic strategies ensuing from information furnished by research. The authors are convinced that the consideration of these concepts would definitely permit the elaboration of optimum and specific treatment for each pediatric patients.

Chapter 1 - A couple of centuries ago, medicine was based on the use of "the right drug for the right disease," to ensure a therapeutic success. Now that we know more about pharmacokinetics, we can say that this statement is totally false. The participation of physicians in the treatment of any disease is not limited just to establishing a good diagnosis and choosing the right drug, but also includes a consideration of the wide individual variability and pharmacokinetic characteristics of the patients as well as to know that therapeutic success can only be achieved by maintaining the therapeutic concentrations at the biological site where the drug exerts its action. Most drugs have a relatively wide therapeutic range however, there are drugs such as diphenylhydantoin, digoxin and gentamicin among others, in which the difference between toxic and therapeutic concentrations is very close. The clinician must know the adverse effects of the drugs and be able to timely identify them. For this, the clinician has to request the plasma concentrations of the drugs. The importance of understanding the pharmacokinetic concepts lies on the above considerations. It is of great value and very basic for the proper management of patients. In this chapter, the authors will discuss the basic pharmacokinetic concepts and their clinical application.

Chapter 2 - During the different stages of life, processes of immaturity, maturity and aging occur, where the body undergoes different changes such as anatomical, physical and biochemical, these processes alter the pharmacokinetics of drugs, together with the individual comorbidities and nutritional status of each patient. It is therefore important to know the pharmacokinetics to individualize medical therapeutics. A fundamental aspect of medicine is medical therapeutics. Unfortunately, only the body weight is considered to administer the dose of a drug, hoping that the therapeutic response is good and similar in different groups of patients, without considering the homeostatic vision of the organism and biological variability. Pharmacological success is evaluated through the empirical test and error criterion, therefore the pharmacological dose is increased or decreased according to the response. It is not generally questioned whether the therapeutic dose is adequate to achieve and maintain plasma levels within the therapeutic range, which is very important to ensure the pharmacological goal. The application of the principles of pharmacokinetics in therapeutic management is important to predict distribution and elimination of drugs in the body through knowledge of plasma concentration curves. The purpose of this chapter is to sensitize the physician and health professionals, to give a better pharmacological management in children.

Chapter 3 - The pediatric age ranges from birth to adolescence and within its chronology, it is divided into periods: newborn, infants, preschool, school, preadolescence and adolescence. During these periods, the child or adolescent must be understood as a subject in development and with constant biological, psychological and social changes, with specific characteristics in each of the stages. The above factors can determine in an important way the health and the onset of diseases. Understanding this is fundamental for any health provider that wants to analyze problems related to childhood. The main causes of illness in patients under 5 years of age are divided into perinatal and postnatal origin. In this chapter, it is intended to address the principal issues leading to postnatal death.

Chapter 4 - LADME refers to the biological pathway which the drugs follow after administration. Such pathway comprises of five processes: liberation, absorption, distribution, metabolism and excretion. Each of the processes is closely related with the therapeutic and toxic effects of a drug. Hence, it is extremely important to take into account the way a drug is administered as well as its pharmaceutical presentation. While most of the references on the study of the pathway have been on adult; in children, the studies performed so far has been very little. Nevertheless, the studies on the topic have recently increased for being considered a crucial area of risk. The present chapter takes a deeper look at the pattern of the profile of LADME process in children.

Chapter 5 - During intrauterine life, the fetus can be exposed to a series of substances ingested by the mother, some of which are necessary for her health but detrimental to the fetus. The noxious effects of such exposure could present in the fetus immediately after exposure or be manifested at the time of delivery and sometimes weeks after birth. The passage of drugs or nutrients across the placenta depends on physicochemical properties of the substances that enable them to cross the placenta barrier, and thus get in contact with the fetus and produce harmful effects. Considering the physicochemical properties of the substances, the possibility of such compounds to cross the placenta barrier and thence to the fetus can be predicted. Equally, it is important to consider the characteristics of the newborn as an immature being, different from adults, when carrying out pharmacokinetic and pharmacodynamic processes. Based on the latter, it is important to know the behavior or characteristics of the fetus and the newborn in the face of drug management and above all, consider the advantages and disadvantages of the use of such drugs for the care of a being yet in development, as described in this work.

Chapter 6 - One of the challenges in the field of pediatric Infectology is how to make a potent antibiotic drug to arrive at the site of infection in active form and inadequate concentration throughout the time required for the drug to exercise its action. In addition, the antibiotic must not interfere with the host´s natural defense mechanism, such as phagocytosis and must be cleared from the body once it has completed its task, since its long-term permanence increases the risk of toxicity. In this chapter, the experience of three clinical cases is presented.

Chapter 7 - Therapeutic drug monitoring (TDM) is an exercise that permits the pediatrician to optimize the regimens of medical treatment in an adequate form, taking into consideration the timely evaluation of the concentrations produced by the administration of a drug as a decisive indicator to adjust the number of doses of the drug and to individualize treatment based on the observed clinical responses as the need arises. In the present report, the authors reviewed the most relevant clinical aspects to carry out TDM. Moreover, the most important pharmacological basis both for the interpretation of concentration values and the values required to effect dose adjustment is analyzed. Likewise, the criteria for the choice of suitable analytical method for the quantification of drug of interest were reviewed. Finally, some recommendations were directed to the physician in order to perform an adequate monitoring that contributes to the clinical-pharmacological control of their patients.

Chapter 8 - Caloric-protein severe malnutrition is a condition in which many nutritional deficiencies simultaneously occur, constituting a public health problem and, in practice, explains the high morbidity and mortality rates in the population of children, especially in developing countries. Approximately one-half of the total population of the world is estimated to have suffered and survived a period of moderate or advanced malnutrition during childhood. It is estimated that about 1000 million children under the age of 15 years who lived in 1980, about 400 million did not receive an adequate diet, because in their societies the same factors that interfere with the correct distribution of available foods prevailed. Due to the effect of malnutrition on the pharmacokinetics of drugs analyzed in this chapter, it is advisable to individualize the therapeutic regimens, to optimize its therapeutic management in pediatric patients principally in those who are under severe malnutrition.

Chapter 9 - Pharmacovigilance (PV) comprises of a series of actions aimed at detecting and registering of Adverse Drug Reactions (ADRs), while pharmacoepidemiology (PE) addresses issues pertaining to all the activities, which involve the detection of drug prescription patterns. The authors describe the procedures of PV and PE of drugs used in a pediatric hospital. The PV activities show that there is a relation between an increase in the incidence of ADRs and the prescription of a larger number of drugs. The PE activities reveal that antibiotics are the most frequently prescribed drugs followed by drugs used for gastrointestinal diseases. Since PV and

PE activities were initiated, they have contributed to an adequate use of drugs in children. When the PE of a hospital is known, drug consumption can be optimally planned. PV and PE demonstrate that when polytherapy is not necessary, it must be avoided. Finally, the present guide can be adopted to initiate PV and PE at any hospital.

Chapter 10 - More than 70% of acute pediatric poisoning is caused by medications. The age group sat the greatest risk of this incident are those between 2 to 5 years and 14 to 18 years, although in this last group, drug ingestion is usually intentional. The purpose of this chapter is to describe the frequency of unintentional drug poisoning in pediatric population, and to review the treatment procedures applied in specific cases. In most of the cases, poisoning is confirmed by determining the plasma concentration of the drug. The most frequent cases of drug poisoning were due to the ingestion of drugs like analgesics mainly acetylsalicylic acid and acetaminophen, antiepileptics, anxiolytics and in lesser proportion other drugs. With the exception of accidental ingestion of drugs, drug poisoning in pediatric population is mainly due to dosing error. Self-medication in this population is unlikely for their age. In most of the cases of unintentional drug poisoning seen in this series, the duration of hospitalization did not exceed 24 hours and no death was registered. Dosing error should be a topic of a major concern for hospitals since this error has been found to be the principal cause of unintentional drug poisoning in infants and young children.

Chapter 11 - Suicide is presently a serious health problem that is seen in different age groups. Most of the children and adolescents that commit suicide have some kind of psychiatric illness and sometimes, small predictors of suicidal ideation are overlooked. Suicidal behavior in children is a delicate topic because in them, it is difficult to predict this behavior. This chapter intends to invite pediatricians, health professionals and authorities to implement actions of alertness to detect factors that could lead to suicide in order to reduce its figures and incidences, especially in pediatric patients.

ACKNOWLEDGMENTS

I express my profound gratitude to Dr. Cyril Ndidi Nwoye Nnamezie for his invaluable contribution in translating this work from Spanish to English and ensuring that the highest language quality standard of the book is maintained. My thanks also go to Dr. Fernanda Reyes Gonzalez for her marvelous technical assistance in the preparation of all the illustrations included in this book. Your contributions have been a great help in bringing this project to a successful end.

Hugo Juarez Olguin

In: The Optimization of Drug Prescribing … ISBN: 978-1-53612-263-3
Editor: Hugo Juarez Olguin

Chapter 1

PHARMACOKINETICS AND ITS CLINICAL APPLICATIONS

***Ismael Lares-Asseff*[1] *and Hugo Juarez Olguín*[2,3,*]**

[1]Centro de Investigación Interdisciplinario para el Desarrollo Integral Regional, Instituto Politécnico Nacional, Durango, Mexico
[2]Laboratorio de Farmacología, Instituto Nacional de Pediatría, Mexico City, Mexico
[3]Departamento de Farmacología, Facultad de Medicina, Universidad Nacional Autónoma de México. Mexico

ABSTRACT

A couple of centuries ago, medicine was based on the use of "the right drug for the right disease," to ensure a therapeutic success. Now that we know more about pharmacokinetics, we can say that this statement is totally false. The participation of physicians in the treatment of any disease is not limited just to establishing a good diagnosis and choosing the right drug, but also includes a consideration of the wide individual variability and pharmacokinetic characteristics of the patients as well as to know that therapeutic success can only be achieved by maintaining the

* Corresponding Author Email: juarezol@yahoo.com

therapeutic concentrations at the biological site where the drug exerts its action. Most drugs have a relatively wide therapeutic range however, there are drugs such as diphenylhydantoin, digoxin and gentamicin among others, in which the difference between toxic and therapeutic concentrations is very close. The clinician must know the adverse effects of the drugs and be able to timely identify them. For this, the clinician has to request the plasma concentrations of the drugs. The importance of understanding the pharmacokinetic concepts lies on the above considerations. It is of great value and very basic for the proper management of patients. In this chapter, we will discuss the basic pharmacokinetic concepts and their clinical application.

INTRODUCTION

The application of pharmacokinetics to clinic has revolutionized the therapeutic management of drugs. Previously, success in therapy for the treatment of human diseases depended, in part, on the physician´s ability to choose the appropriate medication. The training of the physicians and the medical literature were focused on what was called "the pharmacological basis of therapeutics" which was based on the concept of "Right drug for the right illness."

Therapeutic success is possible or likely if the pharmacological properties of a drug can revert or attenuate the pathological process. In many clinical situations, there is a doubt between correct and incorrect drug choice.

With the advent and application of pharmacokinetics in the rational management of drugs in the last years, the criteria for therapeutic management have become enriched. Presently, the concept of "the pharmacological basis of therapeutics" has extraordinarily improved in such a way that the participation of the physician is not limited just only to establish a good diagnosis and to choose the appropriate drug but also to consider individual variability in response to the drugs as well as their pharmacokinetic characteristics. This means that the physician should select the doses of the drug, its route and frequency of administration which would ensure that the right plasma concentrations at the site of biological action are achieved and maintained.

If the concentrations at the site of biological action of a drug are inadequate, the drug may be ineffective, even when it is the right one. Frequently, a drug is discarded for this reason without evaluating first thc therapeutic success through drug monitoring and considering its pharmacokinetic criteria. Moreover, a correct drug can produce toxicity and for that it is discarded without first considering the reasons why it reached elevated concentrations in the organism [1].

Presently, therapeutic success takes into account the relationship between plasma concentrations of a drug and its pharmacological effects. This means that these concentrations are within a safety range or margin i.e., between their therapeutic and toxic concentrations in the receptor site and that they correlate to the therapeutic range of the plasma concentrations of the drug. This range is sometimes called "the therapeutic index." There are, of course, drugs with wide therapeutic index and those with narrow therapeutic index. For the drugs that belong to first group, the relation between the effective minimum concentration and tolerated concentration is broad, while for those with narrow therapeutic index, the relation is very small, therefore it is difficult for the concentration to reach and be maintained within the therapeutic range (figure1).

Penicillins are examples of drugs with wide therapeutic range. Nevertheless, most drugs have relatively wide therapeutic margin but for some drugs listed in table 1.1, the difference between toxic and therapeutic concentrations are very narrow. Therefore, it is obligatory to monitor the doses, the clinical effects and the occurrence of adverse effects of these drugs with narrow therapeutic index and determination of their plasma levels.

The pharmacokinetics of many cardiovascular drugs and anticonvulsive agents, some antibiotics and certain psychotropic drugs, is very importance because their temporal course and intensity of pharmacological action are parallel to their concentrations in some biological fluids.

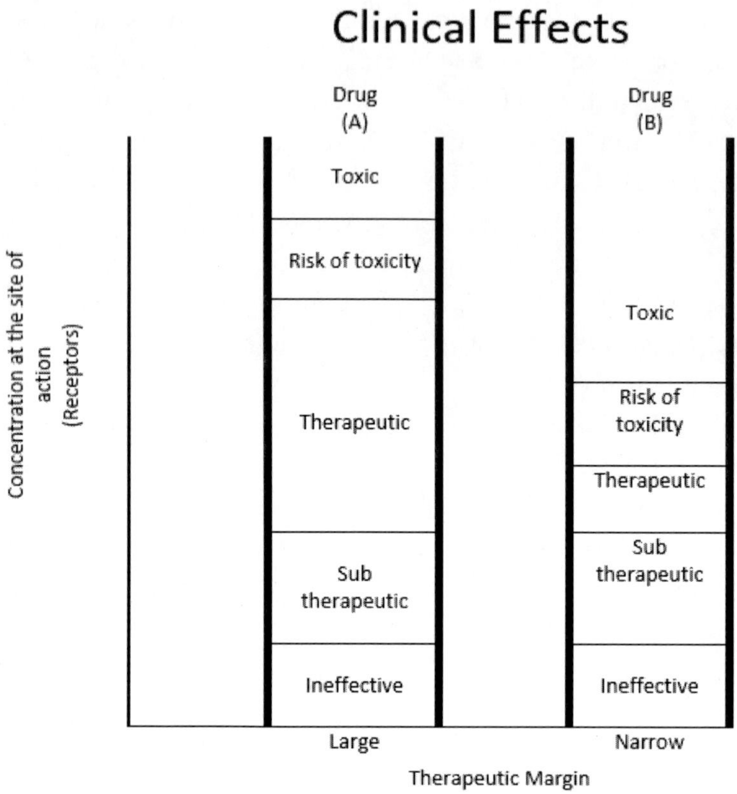

Figure 1. Comparison of the clinical effects of a drug "A" and drug "B" relative to the concentrations at the receptor site.

Table 1. Drugs with narrow therapeutic margin

Drugs with a narrow therapeutic margin
Diphenylhydantoin
Digoxine
Gentamycin
Lithium
Lidocaine
Quinidine
Theophylline

Understanding the pharmacokinetic behavior of these agents and the relationship between their clinical effects and their blood concentrations is very valuable for selecting their appropriate dose regimen and for monitoring their clinical effects. On the other hand, for certain drugs such as antineoplastics, understanding their kinetic behavior may not provide a complete perception of the temporal course of their clinical effects. This is because the net clinical effects of these drugs in the organs are not very important, apparently because of their poor relationship with their plasma concentrations.

PHARMACOKINETIC

Pharmacokinetic is a discipline that uses mathematical model to describe and predict the concentrations and amount of drugs in the body fluids in function of time. Others define it as the study of the time course of a drug and its metabolites in different body fluids, tissues and excreta and the mathematical relationship required to develop models which would permit the interpretation of such data [2]. Thus, the science describing and quantifying the rates of absorption, distribution and elimination of a drug in the organism is called pharmacokinetics.

KINETIC PROCESSES

For conceptual purposes, the behavior of a foreign substance, e.g., a drug, introduced in the body is usually divided into four processes namely absorption, distribution, biotransformation and excretion [3]. Each of these processes is assumed to be independent although, in living organisms they occur simultaneously. In order to understand how the kinetic processes of absorption, distribution and elimination of drugs affect the plasma concentrations, first we must understand the concepts of first-order (linear) and zero-order (non-linear) kinetics.

First-Order Kinetic

The kinetics of a drug are said to be first-order or linear when the rates of absorption, distribution and elimination proportionally change with the changes in the particles of that drug that have not been taken up by the tissues or cells from the blood i.e., the plasma concentrations.

When the values of these concentrations are presented graphically in decimal scale (figure 2), it is evident that as time passes, they become smaller. As the concentrations of a drug decline, its rate of elimination also decreases.

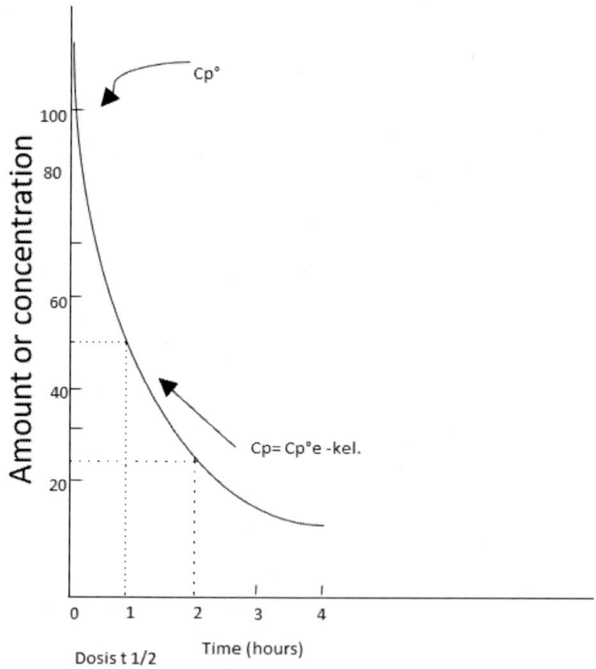

Figure 2. Kinetics of first-order elimination. The amount or concentration of the drug decreases logarithmically in the course of time. The initial plasma amount or concentration produced by a loading dose is Cp°. The half-life time of elimination (t1/2) is the time required to eliminate half of the drug.

When individual plasma drug concentrations are presented on a semi-logarithmic scale (figure 3), the drop in the concentrations is represented by a straight line. It therefore follows that a straight line suggests that changes in the concentration of the drug occur proportionally to the variations in the rate of change of drug concentrations as a function of time (dC/dt).

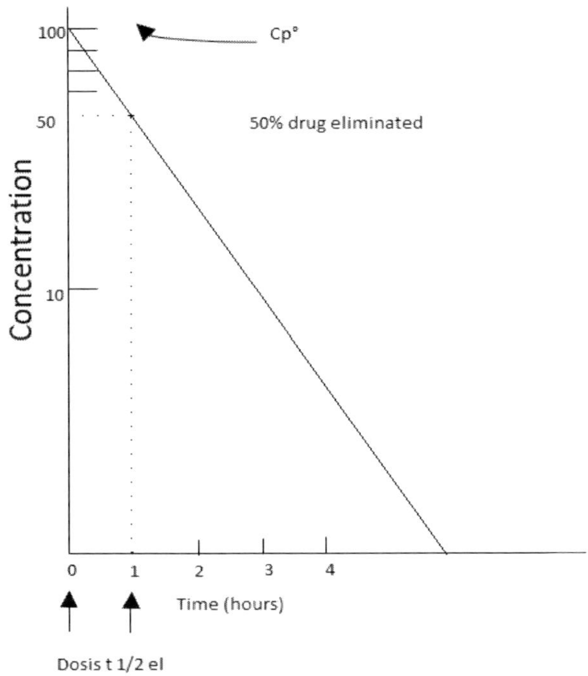

Figure 3. Kinetics of first-order elimination. Plotting the logarithm of concentration versus time produces a straight line. The average lifetime of elimination (t1/2) is the time required for the concentration to decline to half of the original value.

Another way to estimate the kinetics linearity of a drug is by calculating the ratio of the concentration (*C*) at a given time (t) and the dose (D) and then compares this ratio with the calculated ratios obtained at the same time from other doses. For instance,

$$Ct_{500}/D_{500}= Ct_{800}/D_{800}=Ct_{1200}/D_{1200}$$

The kinetics of a drug is dose-dependent, i.e., linear or first-order, when the quotient of the value under the curve of the concentrations as a function of time ($ABCo \rightarrow \alpha$) divided by the dose (D) remains unchanged when the dose increase or decrease [4]. This is evident through the relation:

$$ABCo \rightarrow \alpha_{500}/D_{500} = ABCo \rightarrow \alpha_{800}/D_{800} = ABCo \rightarrow \alpha_{1200}/D_{1200}$$

Zero-Order Kinetics

The elimination of a drug from the body may involve an active process e.g., an enzymatic process (biotransformation). In the event that a drug dose generates high levels of plasma concentrations, the available number of binding sites in the enzyme system may be overstretched or saturated in such a way that the rate of change of the drug concentrations as a function of time (dC/dt) cannot increase at the same rate with which the plasma concentration increase. This means that the drug concentrations increase but without proportional increase in dC/dt.

When the kinetics of a drug is zero-order, the ratio between the concentration at a given time (Ct) or $ABCo \rightarrow \alpha$ and the dose is different [5]. In order to predict the changes in the plasma concentrations as a function of time, it is a fundamental requirement that the kinetics be of first-order. Thus, to correctly interpret the data, it is necessary to first establish if the kinetics is first-order, at least for the dose range used in clinical practice.

Drug Clearance

Clearance is a function of both the intrinsic ability of certain organs (the liver and the kidneys) to excrete or metabolize a drug and the rate of blood flow in them.

In this regard, the venous drug concentration (C_v) will always be less than the arterial concentration (C_a), since some of the drug is eliminated or excreted during the passage of blood through the organs. The rate with which a drug enters an organ is equal to the product of blood flow (Q) and the arterial concentration (C_a) in that organ. The rate at which the drug leaves an organ is equal to the product blood flow and the venous concentration (C_v) in that organ. The difference between the input velocity and output velocity is the elimination rate of the drug by the organ which is calculated as follows:

$$\text{Elimination rate} = Q/C_a\text{-}C_v \quad 1.2$$

The ratio of the elimination rate divided by the input velocity of the drug (Q/C_a) is called the extraction rate (ER). ER is calculated from:

$$ER = Ca\text{-}C_v/C_a \quad 1.3$$

Elimination rate of a drug varies from 0 to 1 depending on how well the organ eliminates or extracts the drug from the blood stream. If the organ eliminates or extracts the drug efficiently, then $C_v = C_a$ and ER = 0. If the organ avidly extracts the drug, that is C_v0, then ER = 1.

By definition, organ clearance (CL) of a drug represents the volume of blood cleaned or purified per unit of time. This can be seen as a constant of proportionality that relates the speed of elimination of a drug with its concentration in the blood as expressed in the following equation:

$$CL = \text{Speed of elimination}/\ C_a \quad 1.4$$

From equation 1.2, we have:

$$CL = Q\ (C_a\text{-}\ C_v/\ C_a \quad 1.5$$

Or from equation 1.3, we have:

$$CL = Q(ER) \quad 1.6$$

Thus, the clearance is equal to the product of blood flow and the rate of extraction. Since the elimination rate is expressed in units of quantity per unit time and the concentration is expressed in units of quantity per unit volume, then clearance is expressed in units of volume per unit of time (mL/min or L/h) which is the same as speed of flow. If the elimination of the drug is a process of first-order, then the clearance is independent of the concentration of the drug.

These equations, which have been developed for single organ, can also be extended to the elimination of the drug from the organism. Thus, the total body clearance of a drug from the blood is equal to the ratio of the total drug elimination rate divided by the concentration of the drug in the blood, where the total elimination rate is the sum of the elimination process that occurs in all the organs.

APPARENT VOLUME OF DISTRIBUTION

The most useful volume term in pharmacokinetics is the apparent volume of distribution at steady state (Vd_{ss}). This represents the proportionality constant which relates the amount of drug in the body at steady state after a sustained venous infusion or repeated administration to the average concentration of the drug at that time. Vd_{ss} is independent of the drug clearance and reflects only the anatomical space occupied by a drug and the relative degree of drug binding in the blood and extravascular space.

Vd_{ss} estimate does not require data obtained at steady state. This distribution parameter can be calculated after a single dose of a drug by means of the following equation [6-8]:

$$Vd_{ss} = dose_{iv} (ABCFM)/(ABC)^2 \quad 1.7$$

where ABCFM is the area under the curve at first moment.

Although equation 1.7 is applied only to intravenous administration, the relation can be easily modified to accommodate the different forms of drug administration. If a drug is administered by intravenous infusion of a short-term [9] at a constant speed, the equation below is used:

$$Vd_{ss} = \frac{\text{Infused doses(ABCFM)}}{ABC^2} = \frac{\text{Infused doses(T)}}{2(ABC)} \qquad 1.8$$

where T is the duration of the infusion. Since the doses infused is equal to Ko T. the equation can also be expressed as follows:

$$Vd_{ss} = \frac{\text{Ko T (ABCFM)}}{ABC2} = \frac{\text{Ko T2}}{2(ABC)} \qquad 1.9$$

MEAN PERSISTENCE TIME

The mean persistence time (MPT) of a drug after the administration of a single dose is given by:

$$MPT = (ABCFM/ABC) \qquad 1.10$$

The MPT of a drug after the administration of an intravenous bolus provides a useful estimate of the time the drug persists in the body and it is closely related to the parameter called elimination half-life. When the drug is rapidly distributed, it can be shown that:

$$MPT_{IV} = 1/K \qquad 1.11$$

where K is the constant rate of first-order.

On considering that the elimination half-life of a drug is equal to 0.693/K which is the time required to eliminate 50% of the dose of the drug administered, then MPT_{IV} tells us the time required to eliminate 63.2% of such dose.

Drug Absorption

The non-compartmental methods for estimating absorption rate of a drug after oral administration are based on the differences in MPT following different methods of administration. In general [8], the following equation is used for this estimation:

$$MTA = MPT_{ni} - MPT_{iv} \qquad 1.12$$

where MTA is the mean time of absorption; MPT_{ni} is the mean persistence time after drug administration in non-instantaneous manner, either orally or intramuscularly; and MPT_{iv} is the mean persistence time following intravenous administration.

Drug Accumulation in Steady State

The steady state (ss) refers to the accumulation of a drug in the body during the administration of multiple doses, when the rate of entry and exit of the drug is equal within a range of doses (figure 4). The extent of the accumulation depends on the elimination half-life of the drug and the dosing interval. In the steady state, the drug concentration oscillates around an average steady state concentration (C_{ss}) with a defined maximum steady state concentration ($C_{ss\ max}$) and minimum steady state concentration ($C_{ss\ min}$) (figure 5). Only in the case of constant infusion rate by intravenous route that the concentrations C_{ss}, $C_{ss\ max}$, and $C_{ss\ min}$ are identical for a drug.

Infusion

Intravenous infusion can be considered as a multiple dose regimen with infinitely small dosing intervals (τ). In figure 6, the curve of blood levels as a function of time for intravenous infusion of a hypothetical drug is shown. The blood levels increase until the plateau or steady state is reached in a time = 5 $t_{½ e}$. At this point, the entry rate is equal to the exit rate. The equation to calculate the steady state concentration (C_{ss}) is as follows:

$$C_{ss} = Vl^0/CL_{total} \qquad 1.13$$

where Vl^0 is the zero-order diffusion rate.

It is obvious that after intravenous infusion, it will take about 5 half-lives before reaching the steady state at the blood level. If one desires an immediate clinical effect, a loading dose at time zero must be administered to immediately reach steady state.

The required infusion rate (Vl^0) is calculated with the following equation:

$$Vl^0 = C_{ss}.CL_{total} \qquad 1.14$$

The required loading dose (LD) to reach the steady state fast is given by the equation:

$$LD = C_{ss}.Vd \qquad 1.15$$

Drug Accumulation in Multiple Doses

The accumulation in case of multiple doses occurs when subsequent drug doses are administered before the previous doses are eliminated. Identical doses (D) are administered in identical dosing intervals (t). The time curve of blood levels will rise with each dose (accumulation) until a steady state is reached depending on the magnitude of the drug´s elimination half-life and the selected dose range (see figure 7). Multiple doses lead to fluctuations in the steady state or plateau levels between $C_{ss\ max}$ and $C_{ss\ min}$ [10].

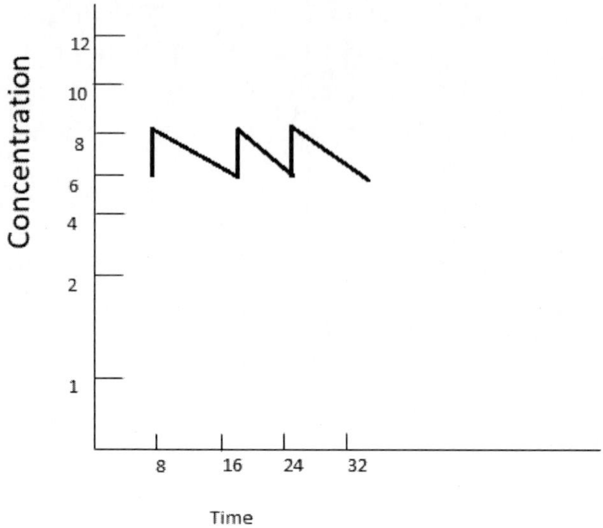

Figure 4. Steady-state concentrations after repetitive administration of a drug which is distributed rapidly with a t ½ el of 12 hours, administered every 8 hours. The proportion of Cmax to Cmin is 1.8.

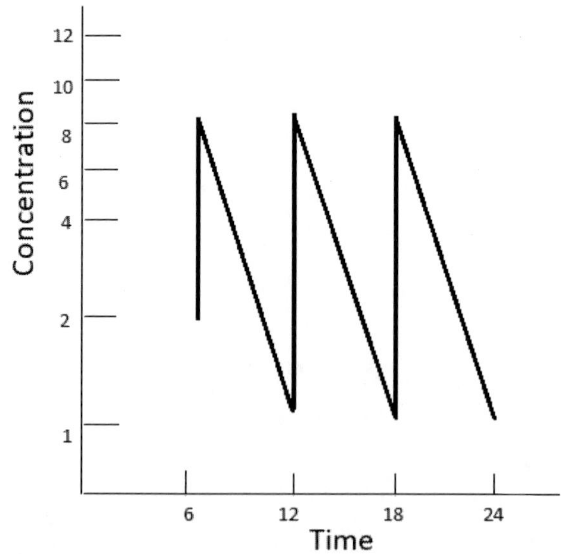

Figure 5. Steady-state concentrations after a repetitive administration of a drug which is distributed rapidly with a t ½ el of 2 hours, administered every 6 hours. The proportion of Cmax to Cmin is 1:7.

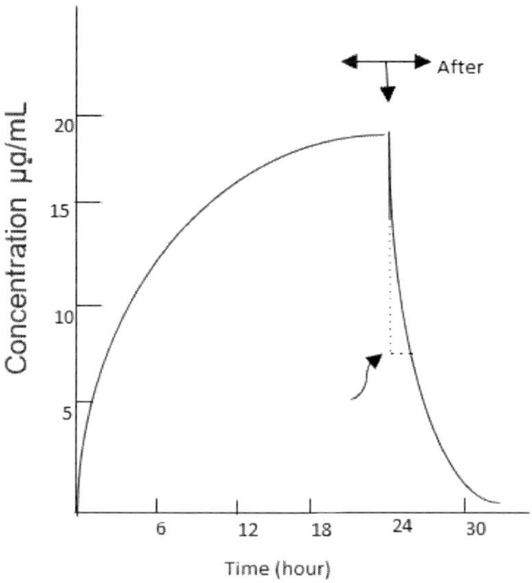

Figure 6.Plasma concentration profile during and after a constant venous infusion of a drug.

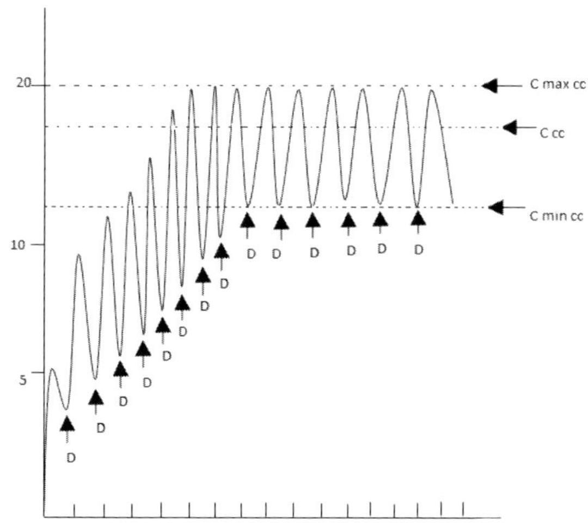

Figure 7. Plasma concentration profile of a drug during oral administrations of repeated of doses at 350 mg every 12 hours. The steady-state maximum plasma concentrations (Cmaxss), the steady-state minimum plasma concentrations (Cminss) and the average steady-state concentration (Css) can be appreciated. D = Dose.

If the identical amount of the doses are administered intravascularly or extravascularly and the drug is completely absorbed, both will result in identical C_{ss}, since the amount administered and absorbed per unit time is the same. Nevertheless, the peaks and the valleys corresponding to the administration will be different and so, will result in smaller fluctuations between $C_{ss\ max}$ and $C_{ss\ min}$.

The mean steady state concentration is calculated with the following equation:

$$C_{ss} = D/CL_{total} \qquad 1.16$$

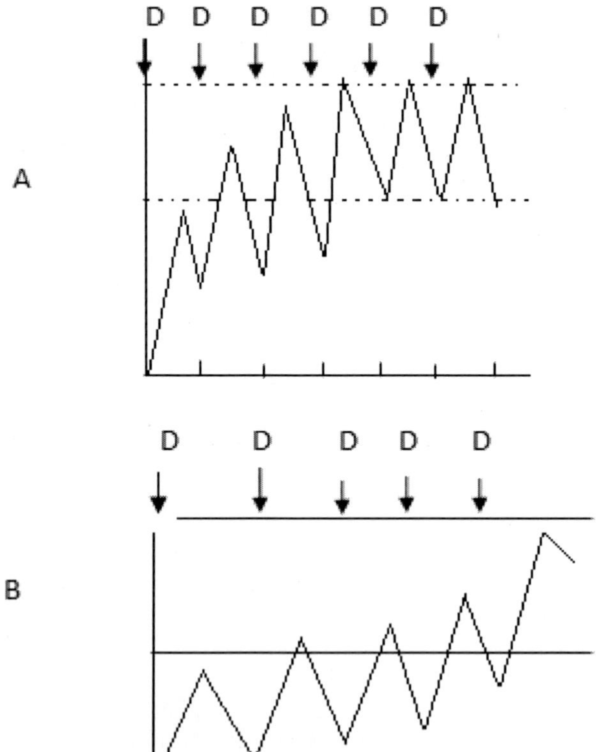

Figure 8. Schematic diagram of a drug during the administration of multiple doses of the same amount but with constant dose range (A) and with dose range (B).

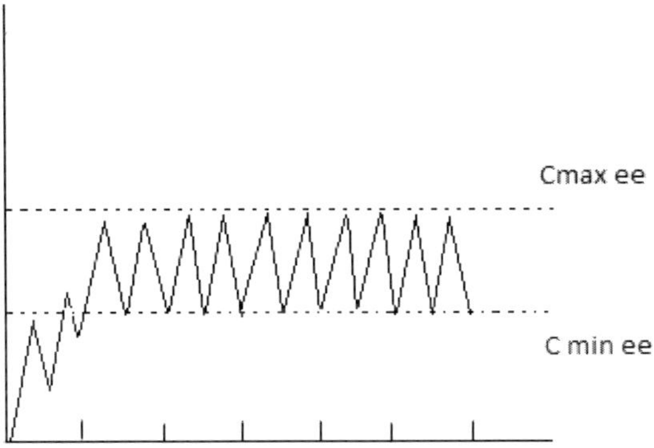

Figure 9. When the dose range is reduced, the equilibrium state is reached fast.

Either by decreasing the dose interval (t) with a constant dose amount (D) or by increasing the dose amount (D) at a constant dose intervals (t), would the blood levels at a steady state increase as can be observed in figure 8. On reducing the dose interval by half, an increase in the steady state concentrations will result with reduced fluctuations between $C_{ss\ max}$ and $C_{ss\ min}$ in blood (figure 9). The mean blood level at steady state is directly proportional to the amount of the dose and inversely proportional to the dose interval. Drug concentrations during the steady state are directly proportional to the amount of the drug absorbed per unit time (D/τ) and the elimination half-life ($t^1\!/\!_2$) of the drug. The time to reach the steady state depends on the elimination half-life. The fluctuations of $C_{ss\ max}$ and $C_{ss\ min}$ between the doses during steady state are proportional to the ratio of dose range and elimination half-life.

Pharmacokinetics Parameters and Their Biological Significance

Body Compartments and Volume of Distribution

The fundamental concepts in pharmacokinetics are the compartments, in that they represent a simplified and useful form to understand the process of drug distribution in the organism. The clinicians should be wary of the interpretations of the pharmacokinetic compartments as these are derived from mathematical calculations rather than from anatomical and physiological aspects.

Although the pharmacokinetic compartments do not correspond to actual anatomic entities, the compartments have numerical dimensions of volume (liters, milliliters, etc.), as if they were the volume of something real. In order to understand the volume of distribution, we have to assume that the drug doses are directly administered into the vascular system.

Drug Distribution

When a drug enters the circulation, its passage or entry into any particular body tissue depends on several factors, such that the physiochemical properties of the drug are of prime importance. Such properties include the molecular size of the drug, the number of charged or polar constituent it contains, its solubility in aqueous or organic medium and its ability to pass through different types of biomembranes.

The distribution of drugs within a tissue depends on both the tissue size and the amount of blood flow in the organs. The concept of compartmental models has been developed to provide a structure that permits to quantify these processes [11].

The Meaning of Biological Half-Life

The characterization of a pharmacokinetic event by the half-life value provides an estimate of the speed with which this process takes place. When the half-life is short, the event proceeds. In contrast, a prolonged half-life indicates a relatively slow process. In many cases, the event is greater than 90% after an interval of four half-lives. Perhaps, the most important of the biological half-life is that it describes the process of elimination or removal of a drug from the body. This half-life of elimination, often abbreviated as $t1/2_{\beta}$, provides knowledge on how quickly a drug will disappear after the administration of a single dose or after the end of a long-term therapy. Like other physiological and pharmacokinetic elements, the rates of elimination of any drug and the values of $t1/2_{\beta}$, varies from person to person and could be deeply influenced by individual factors. Indeed, the half-life of a given drug can vary from time to time even in the same subject [12].

The absorption of a drug is another process that can often be characterized by the half-life values. For virtually all drugs, the absorption occurs much more quickly than the elimination since the values of half-life for absorption are generally much smaller than those corresponding to the elimination half-life.

DESIGN AND ADJUSTMENT OF DOSING REGIMENS AND DOSE ADJUSTMENT

The dosing regimens are designed to achieve or maintain a desired therapeutic concentration at steady state. Such design is based on "average" or "normal" pharmacokinetic parameters and on the desired therapeutic concentrations at steady state [13].

The general approach for designing a dosing regimen is:

1) To select a suitable dose range (τ) in hours. For example 4, 6, 8, 12 and 24 hours, etc. A dose range that is closer to the average half-life time of the drug is often better.
2) To calculate the maintenance dose (MD) using the following equation:

$$MD = C_{ssdesired} . CL_{total} . \tau / F \qquad 1.17$$

where MD is in mg, $C_{ss\ desired}$ is the mean concentration at a steady state expressed in µg/mL, CL_{total}isthetotal clearance of the drug expressed in L/h

(CL_{tot} en L/h = Vd (in L/Kg). Body weight (BW) is expressed in kg. $\beta$is expressed in L x h, while τ is the dose interval expressed in h and F is the fraction of absorbed dose (absolute bioavailability)[14].

$$LD = (1.44\ MD\ t^{1/2})/\tau \qquad 1.18$$

If a maintenance dose will be used, then τ may have to be changed using the following equation

$$\tau = \frac{MD.\ F}{Css.\ CLT} \qquad 1.19$$

This procedure is applicable to all the cases e.g., analgesic, antiarrhythmic, anticoagulant and antidepressant drugs etc., in which the average concentration at steady state is a therapeutic goal.

However for some drugs, the physicians want to reach and maintain minimal inhibitory concentration (MIC) or minimal effective concentration (MEC) throughout the dosing interval or want to reach a final peak concentration during each dosing interval [15]. The first model is usually used for bacteriostatic antibiotics and sulfonamides while the second model is often preferred for bactericidal antibiotics such as penicillins and cephalosporins.

For maintenance dose (MD), according to MIC model and the peak models, the equations 1.26 and 1.27 are used:

$$MD = \frac{Vd.BW.\ MIC\ (1 - e^{-\beta.\tau})}{e\text{-}\beta.\tau.\ F} \qquad 1.20$$

where BW is the body weight.

$$MD = \frac{Vd.BW.\ C_{ssmaxdesired}\ (1 - e^{-\beta.\tau})}{e^{-\beta.\tau max}.\ F} \qquad 1.21$$

In some situations, it would be desirable to maintain a defined MIC in order not to exceed a certain concentration peak in each interval. Such model, called $C_{ssmax} - C_{ssmin}$ model, is frequently used for aminoglycosides [15].

For the method of limited fluctuation or $C_{ssmax} - C_{ssmin}$ where the peak concentrations does not exceed a given value and the valley concentrations are defined by a given value, first the appropriate dosing interval, τ *, (which cannot be freely selected) has to be calculated using the following equation:

$$\tau^* = \left(1\beta.\text{In}\,\frac{C_{ssmax}}{C_{ssmin}}\right) + t_{max} \quad 1.22$$

τ * calculated is then used to calculate MD. Hence we have:

$$MD = \frac{Vd.BW.C_{ss\,max\,desired}\,(1 - e^{-\beta.\tau^*})}{e^{-\beta.\tau max}.\,F} \quad 1.23$$

For all the above examples, the loading dose (LD), which is necessary to immediately achieve the steady state concentrations, is calculated using the equation:

$$MD = \frac{MD}{1 - e^{-\beta.\tau}} \quad 1.24$$

In this case, the method $C_{ssmax} - C_{ss\,min}$ τ^* is used instead of τ.

Any of the dosage regimens designed by one of the methods discussed above or selected by any other method may result in steady state concentration, which is different from the desired concentration. Therefore, the drug concentration must be monitored and if a designated dosage regimen results in a steady state concentration, which is due to the desired concentration, the adjustments can be made as follows[10,16]:

$$\text{New MD} = \frac{C_{ss}\,\text{desired}}{}.\ \text{MD used} \quad 1.25$$

C_{ss} found

or

$$\text{New MD} = \frac{C_{ss}\ \text{max desired}}{C_{ss}\ \text{min found}} \cdot \text{MD used} \qquad 1.26$$

or

$$\text{New MD} = \frac{C_{ss}\ \text{min desired}}{C_{ss}\ \text{min found}} \cdot \text{MD used} \qquad 1.27$$

However, it should be pointed out that the presented equations are very basic since there are more elaborate mathematical calculations that require a vigorous management.

References

[1] Greenblatt, D. J., Shader, R. I. *Pharmacokinetics in clinical practice*. Philadelphia: W.B. Saunders Company, 1985.

[2] Gibaldi, M., Perrier, A. *Pharmacokinetics. J.* Swarbrick ed., New York: Marcel Dekker Inc., 1982.

[3] Zhao, P., Rowland, M., Huang, S. M. Best practice in the use of physiologically based pharmacokinetic modeling and simulation to address clinical pharmacology regulatory questions. *Clin. Pharmacol. Ther.*2012; 92:17-20.

[4] Naranjo, A. C., du Souich, P., Busto, E. U. *Métodos en Farmacologíaclínica.* Programa Regional de Medicamentos Esenciales. Organización Panamericana de la Salud, 1992. [*Methods in Clinical Pharmacology*. Regional Program of Essential Medicines. Panamerican Health Organization, 1992].

[5] Shargel, L., Yu, ABC. *Applied Biopharmaceutics and pharmacokinetics*. Connecticut: McGraw Hill Inc., 2016.

[6] Benet, L. Z., and Galeazzi, R. L. Noncompartmental determination of the steady-state volume of distribution, *J. Pharm. Sci.*1979; 68:1071-1074.The backstory. *AAPS J.*2012.

[7] Samuel, P., Lieberman, S. Simplified method for the long-term study of turnover and body masses of cholesterol by input-output analysis. *Am. J.Clin. Nutr.* 1974; 27:1214-20.

[8] Laurberg, P. Mechanisms governing the relative proportions of thyroxine and 3,5,3'-triiodothyronine in thyroid secretion. *Metabolism* 1984; 33:379-92.

[9] Varughese, A., Brater, D. C., Benet, L. Z., Lee C. S. Ethambutol kinetics in patients with impaired renal function. *Am. Rev. Respir. Dis.* 1986; 134:34-8.

[10] Turnheim, K. Drug dosage in the elderly. Is it rational? *Drugs Aging*.1998; 13:357-79.

[11] Collier, P. S. Some considerations on the estimation of steady state apparent volume of distribution and the relationships between volume terms. *J. Pharmacokinet. Biopharm.* 1983; 11:93-105.

[12] Liu, D. Y. Dosage regimen maintaining a plateau level of drugs for intravenous injection. *Hua Xi Yi Ke Da Xue Xue Bao* 1987; 18:148-52.

[13] Iliadis, A., Bruno, R., Cano, J. P. Dynamical dosage regimen calculations in linear pharma-cokinetics. *Comput. Biomed. Res.* 1988; 21:203-20.

[14] Segre, G. Relevance, experiences, and trends in the use of compartmental models. *Drug Metab. Rev.* 1984; 15:7-53.

[15] Dorokhov, V. V., Kholodov, L. E. Analysis of the relation between pharmacokinetic processes and pharmacological effects in humans. *Farmakol. Toksikol.*1985; 48:119-25.

[16] Ritschel, W. A. *Graphic approach to clinical pharmacokinetic*, 2nd ed. Chapter II, J.R. Barcelona: Prous Publishers, 1984; 13-17.

In: The Optimization of Drug Prescribing … ISBN: 978-1-53612-263-3
Editor: Hugo Juarez Olguin

Chapter 2

PHARMACOKINETIC, GROWTH AND DEVELOPMENT

***Ismael Lares-Asseff*[1,*] *and Gabriela Pérez Guille*[2]**
[1]Centro de Investigación Interdisciplinario para el Desarrollo Integral Regional, Instituto Politécnico Nacional, Durango, México
[2]Laboratorio de Farmacología,
Instituto Nacional de Pediatría, Mexico City, Mexico

ABSTRACT

During the different stages of life, processes of immaturity, maturity and aging occur, where the body undergoes different changes such as anatomical, physical and biochemical, these processes alter the pharmacokinetics of drugs, together with the individual comorbidities and nutritional status of each patient. It is therefore important to know the pharmacokinetics to individualize medical therapeutics. A fundamental aspect of medicine is medical therapeutics. Unfortunately, only the body weight is considered to administer the dose of a drug, hoping that the therapeutic response is good and similar in different groups of patients, without considering the homeostatic vision of the organism and

* Corresponding Author Email: ismaelares@yahoo.com

biological variability. Pharmacological success is evaluated through the empirical test and error criterion, therefore the pharmacological dose is increased or decreased according to the response. It is not generally questioned whether the therapeutic dose is adequate to achieve and maintain plasma levels within the therapeutic range, which is very important to ensure the pharmacological goal. The application of the principles of pharmacokinetics in therapeutic management is important to predict distribution and elimination of drugs in the body through knowledge of plasma concentration curves. The purpose of this chapter is to sensitize the physician and health professionals, to give a better pharmacological management in children.

WHY CLINICAL PHARMACOKINETIC RESEARCH IN PEDIATRICS?

No matter the specialty, physicians are constantly facewith the problem of the therapeutic management of their patients. Unfortunately, it is not alwaysquestioned whether the chosen dose is adequate to reach and maintain the plasma level within the therapeutic interval, which is quite pertinent to ensure pharmacological success.

To date, the prescription of drugs is based on the homeostatic vision of the organism and/or the function of the dynamic changes that determine the biological variability that may be compromised within the ranges of normality and which precisely reflects great adaptability and flexibility of various biological functions. Usually, the physician assumes that the dose of a drug, calculated on the basis of body weight, is equally effective in different individuals and that the therapeutic response is independent of the time in which it is administered.

Pharmacological success is evaluated according to the empirical test and error criterion. Hence, based on the pharmacological response, the dose of a drug is increased or reduced without knowing the changing dynamics of the organism, which becomes evident even in the same subject, in different circumstances and hours of his or her life. Scientific and technological advances of diagnostic and therapeutic resources in the last three decades are overwhelming and represent a challenge to the physician. Somehow, the physician has to accept and manage the knowledge and current resources in this regard in the clinical practice. If the physician is left behind in this knowledge, apart from trying to avoid putting into use these new scientific resources to improve the diagnosis, treatment, timely detection of disease risk and death of his patient, he would remain marginalized in the universal knowledge.

Advancement of various disciplines such as clinic pharmacology, biopharmacy, biomathematics, physiology, and recently the development of analytical chemistry, has facilitated the application of analytical techniques in the quantification of drug levels in biological fluids even in extraordinarily small concentrations.

Recently, pharmacokinetic application and the use of computers in clinical practice have modernized the therapeutic management of the patients thus, improving the efficacy and safety of drug use. For optimal administration of drugs, it is completely pertinent to know the mechanisms of absorption, distribution and elimination as well as the kinetics of these processes that constitute pharmacokinetic.

The application of pharmacokinetic principles in the management of patients is the work of clinical pharmacokinetics. Hence, the aim of this discipline is to predict the distribution and elimination of drugs in the body through the knowledge of drug plasma concentration declination curves. This will permit physicians to evaluate and design, in a more rational way, the therapeutic regimens of drugs. When the pharmacokinetic parameters of a patient are known, the physician will be in a position to interpret how the body of a patient is handling the administered drug. Pharmacokinetic parameters are indicators of the changing dynamic of physiological processes that take part in the degradation and excretion of a drug. For instance, they bring into evidence the speed of absorption, distribution and elimination of an administered drug; the amount of it that is still existing and the overall length of time it stays in the body as well as the speed with which it is distributed in different body compartments, the volume of body fluids for its distribution and the concentration of the same. By having this knowledge, a physician is in a position to design a dosing regimen so as to achieve the therapeutic objective in a more precise way.

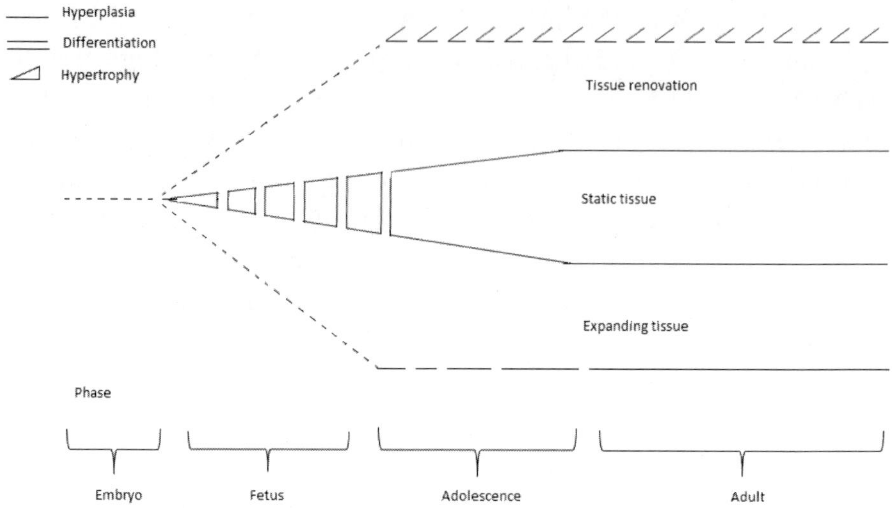

Figure 1. Alternative route of growth and differentiation of tissues and organs. Tissue renewal with long life proliferation. The static tissues permanently lose the ability to differentiate as in the early stage of life. Consequently, they engage only in expansive growth. The tissues in expansion do not suspend their division until there is a stop in body growth, a time when they are completely differentiated.

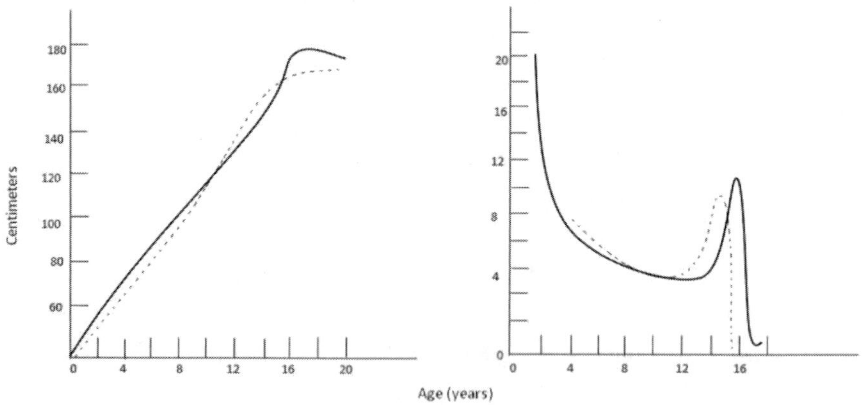

Figure 2. Growth in supine length and height (cm) of boys (continuous line) and girls (intermittent line) (left Figure). Speed of growth (cm/year) in supine longitude and height (right Figure).

As part of the processes of immaturity, maturity and aging, that characterize the different life stages, the body undergoes anatomical, physical-biochemical and body composition changes (Figure 1) as well as a great number of physiological changes that may alter, in a dramatic form, drug bioavailability and use by the body.

Physiological processes determining drug availability in the body undergo radical changes during biological maturity. At the same time, the processes of absorption, distribution, metabolism and excretion are modified during the different life stages– newborn, babies, infants or toddlers, preschool, school, teens, teenage or adolescence, adult and old age – as a consequence of determined changes due to growth and increase in the speed of the same (Figure 2). These changes define 3 characteristics in pediatric therapies and in old-aged people:

1) The stages of childhood and old age (senescence) are the extreme periods of human life that represent high risk stage in drug management due to evolution and involution processes that characterize them.
2) Drug availability changes during the processes of growth, development and aging.
3) Interindividual variability is not an exception in drug availability but a rule since it has been observed in a great number of drugs. This variability is determined by sex, nutritional status, diet, circadian rhythms, smoking, disease status, drug-drug interactions as well as age and other factors.

All these elements require the participation of the physician in order to enrich his clinical experience with the application of pharmacokinetic and drug monitoring in clinical practice as part of the modernity in therapeutic management that will lead to a more scientific drug therapy.

The experience gained from the clinical observations as well as in pharmacokinetic quantification will provide an extraordinary field to conjugate clinical research with basic research for the benefit of sick people.

Clinical Pharmacokinetic in the Management of Patients

Pharmacokinetic is a branch of pharmacology and a term coined up by F. H. Dots in 1953, [1] and literally means the application of kinetic to pharmakon, a Greek word for drugs and poisons. Kinetic is a branch of knowledge involving the changes or movement of one or more variables as a function of time. The application of this discipline in clinical practice is known as "clinical pharmacokinetic." The primary purpose of pharmacokinetic is to study the temporal course of drug concentrations or amount and its metabolites in biological fluids, tissues and excreta as well as its pharmacological response and construction of an appropriate model to interpret the data [2].

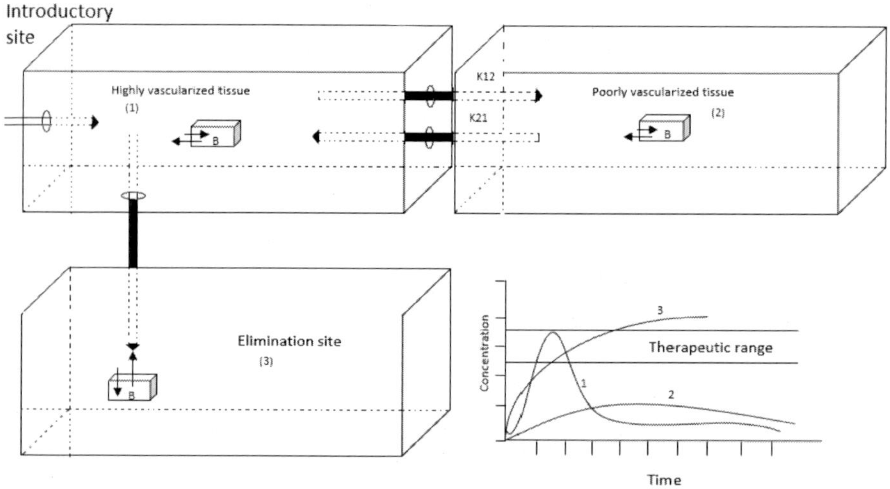

Figure 3. Theoretical model that conceive the organism as a multi-compartmental system, constituted by a central compartment divided into deep tissues (1), poorly vascularized tissues (2) and elimination sites (3). As can be seen, there are bidirectional transference rates between the compartments. The concentration of the drug in function of time in the different compartments is shown in the lower right graph.

Pharmacokinetic data obtained experimentally from human or from animal model are analyzed using theoretic models with mathematical representations of a part or of the organism as a whole (Figure 3). Hence, as Wager [3], pointed out, the purpose of pharmacokinetic to reduce the data to a number of biologically significant parameters and to use such parameters to also predict the results of a study in a patient, which in addition from being too expensive, took a long time. Another definition was given by Gibaldi and Levy [4] who indicated that pharmacokinetic is the study and characterization of the temporal course of absorption, distribution, metabolism and excretion of a drug and the relation of these processes to the intensity and the temporal course of the therapeutic and adverse effects of the drug. The fast growth of pharmacokinetics during the last two decades has been possible, thanks to the analytical method, that has allowed the measurement of drug concentrations even in extremely small amount as well as its application in medical therapy as a tool to improve, in a rational way, therapeutic medicine.

The future of pharmacokinetic in the care of the patients includes among others:

1) Individualization of the treatment regimen
2) Use of pharmacokinetic parameters like variables to guide the synthesis, development of new drugs for therapeutic use and the clinical trials for the approval of new quimiotherapeutical agents.
3) Development and use of non-invasive methods to evaluate the concentrations of drugs in the patients.
4) Determination of intra and interindividual variability of pharmacokinetic parameters.
5) Aids in the determination of mechanisms of drug interactions and how to avoid them.
6) The use of pharmacokinetic as a diagnostic tool allows the determination of the elimination capacity of the organism.
7) Estimation of populationalpharmacokinetic parameters and their variability which may help in the therapeutic management of the patients.

8) Evaluate already established treatment regimen and provides the essential elements to design a more adequate treatment regimen from pharmacokinetic data in a particular biological and physiological reality.

Its purpose is then to calculate and predict optimal dosing regimen that is both effective and safe.

In Whom Should a Pharmacokinetic Study Be Performed?

Pharmacokinetic knowledge, from an ethical and therapeutic point of view, is necessary for every patient that will be indicated a treatment regimen in chronic form or in patients who have been indicated a regimen of treatment in shorter periods of time with a very toxic drug or a drug with a very narrow index or therapeutic window where the relation between the maximum tolerated concentration and the minimum effective concentration is very small. Moreover, the pharmacokinetic study should be performed in every subject that will receive medications, whose half-life elimination time (*t ½ el*) is very short as well as in every severe patient receiving multiple medications without minding if they have functional impairment of the most important organs involved in drug elimination. Therefore, pharmacokinetic study must be performed in order to know the parameters that would enable the diagnosis in the way in which the organism handles a determined medication and aid in making a therapeutic design that takes into account the changing dynamic characteristics of the organism in diseased state.

Evaluation of Drug Concentrations in the Organism

With the objective to properly characterize the decay of a given dose of medicine, after intravenous administration or by any other route, to an experimental animal or to an individual, normally in different time intervals previously established for the medicine, the blood concentrations of the medicine are determined. It could be observed that once the medicine reaches a maximum concentration, it gradually decreases in a peculiar way with respect to time. When the medicine is intravenously administered, at first, the rate of this decrease is fast and later with a slower rate (Figure 4). In this case, the mathematical deductions lead to the conclusion that the disappearance process of the medicine fits into a mathematical equation that defines the kinetic behavior [5]:

$$Cp = Co.\ e^{kel.t} \qquad \text{(Eq. 1)}$$

where Cp is drug blood concentration at different times after the administration, Co equals the plasma concentration at time zero once the slope of elimination phase is extrapolated to the axis of the ordinates. The value *e* is the base of natural logarithms which is raised to power *–kel.t* where *t* represents the time elapsed and *Kel*, the elimination rate constant and corresponds to the value of the slope which is unique for each drug and reflects the organism´s biotransformation capacity to eliminate the drug.

The very nature of equation 1 allows its transformation to a straight line when it is logarithmically expressed either by substituting natural logarithm on both sides of the equation:

$$Ln\ Cp = LnCo - Kel.t \qquad \text{(Eq. 2)}$$

or with base logarithms 10(log)

$$Log\ Cp = Log\ C.\ Kel.\ t/2.303 \qquad \text{(Eq. 3)}$$

On representing the equations in semilogarithmic form and the time in ordinal form, the data are adjusted to a straight line (Figure 5). The slope of the line of fall of the drug concentrations directly gives us its elimination constant *Kel* that represents the fraction of the drug eliminated per unit of time.

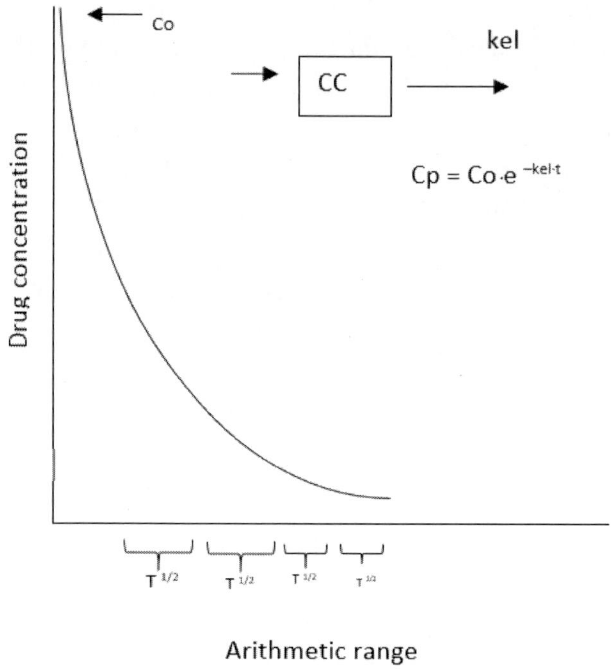

Figure 4. Graph describing the plasma concentration decay curve of a drug with respect to time. In this case, the data are presented in an arithmetical scale.

Due to the particular characteristics of the process, two phases as illustrated in Figure 6 can be defined and these correspond to the sections of a broken line – the first section (a) of the broken line of the Figure corresponds to simultaneous processes of distribution and elimination, while the section (b) of the same line describe the elimination process, which is slower.

The equation which will describe the different blood drug concentration values in this case is more complex since it will be defined by two exponential phases as follows:

$$Cp = Ae^{at} + Be^{bt} \quad \text{(Eq. 4)}$$

where A corresponds to the intercept in the ordinate of the extrapolated line (a), B to the intercept of the extrapolation of the line (b), while the alpha and beta values correspond to the constants of distribution and elimination rates respectively. This type of kinetic is known as bi-exponential or bi-compartmental because it corresponds to two compartment open model (TCOM) [6].

In very rare occasions, decay curves that correspond to multi-compartmental models (three or more compartments) which are used to define the changes that are described by complex poly exponential equations are observed. When a medicine is orally administered, the kinetic behavior apart from corresponding to what is described above extends the absorption process, which comprises of the amount of drug absorbed, the peak and the absorption time as well as the rate of absorption.

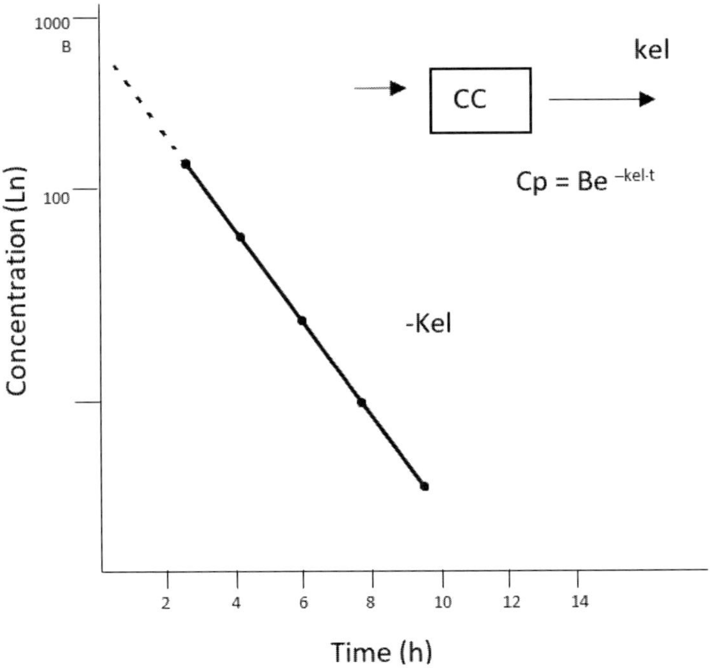

Figure 5. On plotting the experimental concentrations of a drug as a function of time using a semi logarithmic scale, it enables the definition of the compartmental model which in this case corresponds to one-compartmental open model (OCOM) in virtue of the fact that kinetic reaction is the first order for presenting a linear slope which in this case is negative with t1/2 representing the elimination half-life.

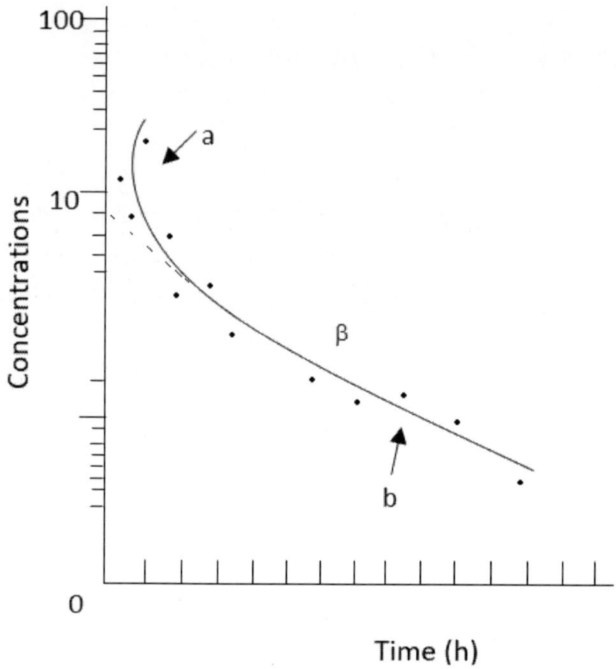

Figure 6. Graph describing the curve of drug concentration decline as a function of time and which when plotted in a semilogarithmic scale presents two exponential phases. The first phase corresponds to fast distribution (a) and the second (b) with a slower declination represents the elimination.

PHARMACOKINETIC PARAMETERS

Pharmacokinetic parameters are simplified values that are obtained from the decay curves of plasma concentrations in biological fluids as a function of time and represent it in a practical and simplified way, the different kinetic processes of absorption, distribution, biotransformation and excretion of a determined medicine. Therefore, pharmacokinetic parameters reflect the dynamic behavior of a specific medicine that will be defined by a determined dose in an individual under certain biological or physiological conditions and at a determined hour. They could, as well, be genetically determined or subject to environmental changes with high probability of presenting intra and interindividual variations hence, they reflect a dynamic process that is developed over a determined time under certain biological and environmental conditions that most of the times are not valid for the same individual when his physiopathological conditions change.

Table 1. Formulas to calculate the pharmacokinetic parameters

For one-compartment open model	For two-compartment open model
t1/2 el = 0.69.3/Kel	t1/2β = 0.693/β
Vd = D/Cpo	Vdβ = D/ A+B
Cl_T = Kel.Vd	CL_T = βVd

Cl_T = total body clearance, Vd = volume of distribution, Kel = the constant of elimination rate of OCOM (value of the slope), A = extrapolated interchange value of the distribution value, B = the extrapolated value of the intercept of the elimination phase, Cp = time zero, plasmatic concentration, β = the elimination rate constant of TCOM (value of the slope in the terminal phase).

From a practical point of view, pharmacokinetic parameters, depending on the process studied, represent the capacities, rates, volumes and times of elimination of a drug which will permit the description interpretation and quantification of the studied phenomenon. When pharmacokinetic parameters are available, it is possible to design a treatment regimen in a rational way using the pharmacokinetic knowledge, which is based on the quantification of the capacities of absorption, distribution and elimination of a medicine in a particular individual.

The pharmacokinetic parameters required to design or redesign a new treatment regimen are directly obtained from the slope of the curve of the medicine measured at different times. Once the zero time (extrapolated value), as well as the value of the slope of the corresponding terminal phase of the elimination process, which represents the constant of elimination rate (Kel) of the medicine are available, the kinetic parameters required for designing the dose can be obtained from these values without minding if the data have been adjusted to a mono or biexponential model. The choice of the formulas to calculate the pharmacokinetic parameters are shown in Table 1.

Effects of Disease Status on Pharmacokinetic

The state of the disease can modify the number of kinetic parameters that alter the concentrations at a steady state. The ability to predict or understand the way in which pathological conditions can modify drug, kinetics requires an understanding of the interrelationship of the different parameters. Metabolic clearance is the most critical parameter in designing dosage regimen of drugs and it the most easily calculated and used method. For drugs that follow a first order kinetic process, the clearance can be calculated independently of the number of compartments, by using the measurements of the area under the curve. During the steady state, the clearance can be calculated from dose rate and average concentration measured in the steady state by the following formula:

$$Dose\ rate = Cl_T.Css \qquad \text{(Eq. 5)}$$

where Cl_T corresponds to clearance and Css to average concentration at steady state.

Therefore:

$$Cl_T = dose\ rate.Css \qquad \text{(Eq. 6)}$$

The body clearance does not have the same ambiguities associated with the volume of distribution and the different half-lives that characterize multi-compartment pharmacokinetic models. Nevertheless, these parameters have to be estimated if one wishes to characterize the temporal course of the plasma concentrations of a drug when administering intermittent doses, particularly the expected minimum and maximum steady state concentrations. It is extremely important to determine and characterize the pharmacokinetic behavior of medicines, above all, in subjects that present important pathophysiological changes and who require a poly-pharmaceutical medical management.

Pharmacokinetic During Growth and Development

An organism reaches growth only after successfully completing a continuous series of intricate and elaborate events. The sequence starts with the conception followed by the processes of growth and development that progress in a predictable way. The sequence is also associated with a wide variety of physiological functions, many of which vary in proportion with the weight and the body surface. These have been the acceptable bases to adjust the doses of drugs for individuals of different sizes and ages in such a way that the extrapolation of adult doses to organisms in development has resulted in unexpected toxic effects in some cases.

In all developmental studies, basing the prescription on scientific data obtained from a particular age group gives way to a poorly safe and effective administration. The possibility of treating fetal diseases with the medicines administered to the mother is a perspective which will only be achieved when the pharmacokinetic of different compounds are precisely characterized in the unit mother-placenta-fetus.

Pharmacokinetic: Basic Principles

Therapeutic agents administered to living organisms undergo a series of changes which eventually condition their interaction with specific receptors and production of pharmacological effects. Once the drug is absorbed, it enters the vascular system and circulates both in free form and bound to plasma protein. By these means, it is distributed in the entire organism. The effects of the medicine will appear when it begins to eliminate by both the hepatic biotransformation and renal excretion.

After oral administration, absorption is a phenomenon that is influenced by the special characteristics of the drug like:

1) The dissolution rate of the medicine which largely depends on its solubility in water and the degree of ionization. However, for the changes associated with age, factors of the host and his peculiarities become important in this aspect. For instance, the absorption will be influenced by gastrointestinal content, pH, intestinal motility, gastric emptying time and the mesenteric blood flow.
2) Drug distribution is governed by other elements that influence lipid solubility, the degree of ionization and the binding properties of the drug to the plasma proteins and specific tissues as well as other routes like saliva, feces, bile and sweat.

Although the above steps are carried out in all developmental studies, there are many qualitative and quantitative differences. Maturity implies continuous changes that first occur in a very complex unit constituted by the mother, placenta and fetus, and later in the newborn like a single individual who is adapted to extra uterine life.

THE MOTHER

Pregnancy produces many physiological changes in the organism which influence on the effect and disposition of medications [7]. Changes in oncotic pressure (20% in the last trimester), as well as the gradual increase in total water content and in blood volume modify the distribution of drugs. For instance, the relative hypoalbuminemia of the third trimester of pregnancy is responsible for the decrease in drug protein binding capacity as occurs in the case of sulfisoxazole [8].

The renal function is changed during pregnancy and this is reflected in renal excretion rate seen in the increase in glomerular filtration rate as well as in changes in tubular reabsorption capacity. During late pregnancy, changes in body position will affect renal excretion of foreign compounds as was demonstrated by a decrease in urine volume and clearance of insulin and paraminohipurate in supine position.

The metabolic capacity also undergoes some changes during pregnancy. The mechanisms explaining these changes during pregnancy is unclear, but may not be related to hormonal changes such as increased amount of reduced progesterone derivatives. These can exert an inhibitory action on the activity of certain drug metabolizing enzymes [9].

THE FETUS

When a medicine is administered to a mother, it reaches the organism of the fetus after crossing the placenta. Exposure of the fetal tissue to the drug will depend on the kinetic equilibrium between the maternal blood and fetal blood and on the distribution within the fetus.

The fetus has several forms of theoretical absorption, although not necessarily in classicsense, since drugs are transferred from the maternal-fetal circulation. For instance, the fetus drinks from 5 to 70 ml of amniotic fluid per hour and the amount of drug present in the gut will depend on its concentration. For some drugs excreted through the kidney, the active enzyme B-glucuronidase present in the intestinal mucus permits the reabsorption and thus drug recirculation. Another route of theoretical absorption is through the fetal skin which appears to be permeable to water and probably to other substances, including drugs.

Distribution of Drugs

Body composition varies with fetal growth. Total body water decreases from approximately 76% at birth which reflects a decrease in the amount of extracellular fluid. Thus, water-soluble drugs have a larger volume of distribution in early developmental studies. In contrast, lipid-soluble drugs such as diazepam and thiopental vary in their distribution depending on their fat content. In the fetus, the amount of fat is minimal which begins to be deposited in the third month of intrauterine life.

With respect to the binding capacity of drugs to plasma proteins, there are differences both in qualities and quantities. It appears that the fetal proteins are less effective than that of the newborn.

Metabolism

The fetus uses the placenta as the main organ of expression. Nevertheless, from the fetal stage, the metabolic pathways become evident, which through the enzymatic activities facilitate the transformation of drugs in compounds that can be excreted more easily. Oxidation is a biotransformation route which involves electron transport that uses cytochrome p450 as the final step. The components of this chain have been measured in human fetal liver and when they are expressed per gram of tissue present in the liver microsomal preparation, they resulted to have a similar amount in both fetus and adult. Early experimental works indicate that the oxidizing amount was evident for endogenous substrates and not for xenobiotic compounds. The metabolizing activity of the drugs is not only found in the fetal liver but also in an important proportion in the fetal adrenal tissue which exhibits a high concentration of cytochrome p450. In recent years, it has been shown that the enzymatic activity may be significantly increased by the administration of certain medications which constitute the process known as drug induction and which has had an important clinical application. The opposite phenomenon of inhibition of drug metabolism has to be visualized in the same way [10-11].

Excretion

The fetus uses the maternal organism as the main route of excretion of foreign compounds. The drugs are transferred through the placenta in opposite direction. The fetal kidneys produce urine during the last trimester of pregnancy and contribute in an important way in the production of amniotic liquid in which the drugs and metabolites of both maternal and fetal origin can be measured.

THE NEWBORN

Birth implies a series of anatomical and physiological changes in the newborn, which are pertinent for its adaptation in the new external environment. Therefore, the management of drugs by the organism in this stage is performed differently than in later stage of life.

Absorption

It is indisputable that the morphological and physiological changes of digestive tract modify the absorption of medicines. At birth, there are some changes in bacterial colonization and rapid alterations in the splenic circulation. The available surface area will influence the rate and extent of absorption. The gastrointestinal tract of the newborn represents a larger portion than in the later stages of life. It seems that intestinal permeability is increased since the passage of molecules of intact protein has been observed in early stages of life. Gastrointestinal absorption of drugs is regulated by 2 factors: pH-dependent diffusion and the time of gastric emptying, both of which undergo continuous changes after birth. For instance, the gastric pH is within the neutral range at birth and falls from the values of 1.0 to 3.0 in the first 24 hours, in such a way that in the next 9 days, a relativelyachlorhydria is presented. At 3 years of age, the gastric pH values become equal to that of an adult.

The low gastric acidity explains the low concentrations of some drugs in newborn infants, when compared with that obtained in older children [12-13]. The time of gastric emptying varies also with the age. It is slower in the newborn than in the adult, a situation which continues until 6 months of age. Although bowel movements are irregular and unpredictable, it can be modified by diet and feeding schedules [14]. In the case of intramuscular or subcutaneous administration of drugs, the absorption rate will depend on regional blood flow which changes during the first two weeks of life. There are variations in the relative blood flow to different muscle groups and these could be intensified under hypoxic conditions.

Distribution

The total body water, extracellular water and intracellular water are compartments in which the drugs are distributed. The total body water is much bigger in the newborn and varies from 85% of body weight in preterm infants to 70- 75% in term infants and reaches 60% at the age of one year. In contrast, the volume of extracellular space is approximately 40 - 45% of the body weight and 15% in adult. These changes reflect that the intestinal volume and the plasmatic compartment remain relatively constant, with 4 to 5% of body weight throughout the life. The intracellular space increases from 34% at birth to 43% at 3 months of age. Thereafter, it goes down until it reaches a value similar to that of the newborn. Between the first and third year of life, all the compartments increase and then gradually decline to adult values. The fat content is 1% lower in preterm infants than in a term child with 15%.

In plasma, drugs bind mainly to albumin. Such binding depends fundamentally on the drug structure and nature of binding formed with the protein. This could be affected by qualitative and quantitative changes in the plasma proteins as well as by competition with endogenous or exogenous compounds for the binding sites. Even when term children have plasma albumin in a value equivalent to that of adults, the total proteins and plasma protein binding get to adult values at one year of age. The differences in protein bindings between newborns and adults can be determined not only by the lower concentration of plasma proteins but also by the qualitative differences in the binding properties. For instance, some endogenous substances may occupy binding sites during the first days of life thus, reducing the binding capacity [15-16].

There are a number of pharmacokinetics studies that bring into evidence all the above mentioned, inconsequently, the fraction of free circulating drug increases. On the contrary, in view of the reduced fat content in the newborn and the high lip solubility of diazepam, its distribution is lower [17].

Metabolism

Newborns seem to have limited capabilities for drug biotransformation for possessing the low activity of enzymes responsible for the function of mixed oxidation and conjugation with glucuronides which could be compensated by the mechanism of adequate sulfation. The maturation rate of the different metabolic pathways seems to be similar as demonstrated by different studies. Decreased activity of the oxidative pathway in newborns has been demonstrated in studies involving several drugs [18].

A decreased capacity to form hydroxylated metabolites of diazepam and mepivacaine was found in children. In addition, the half-life elimination of these compounds in newborns is more prolonged than in premature infants [19]. Conjugation ability was studied for p-aminobenzoic acid, which is coupled to glucuronic acid and p-aminophenol (the oxidized metabolite of Acetanilide) which is glucuronidated before being excreted. The study revealed that the elimination half-lives were more prolonged in preterm infants than in more mature infants, although the difference disappeared at 3 months of life [20-21]. It is feasible that the metabolizing activity of drugs is modified by environmental factors as is the case of drug administration or as is the case of drugs which when administered chronically determines self-induction in their biotransformation [22-23].

Excretion

Kidney anatomy and function change with the age. The majority of the glomeruli are present at the end of 36 weeks of gestational age and the postnatal changes occur only in the elongation and maturation of the tubules of some of the nephrons. This indicates that a term newborn has a structural integrity in contrast to those born prematurely with the probability of having a deficiency in the immature tubules and glomeruli. Most of the medicines administered, whether metabolized or unchanged, are eliminated from the organism by renal excretion [24].

The importance of glomerular filtration maturity in drug elimination is exemplified by the group of aminoglycoside antibiotics, which are excreted unchanged. Their elimination half-lives in preterm infants are longer than in older children. Drugs that depend on tissue secretion such as penicillin G and a good number of semisynthetic penicillins are slowly eliminated by the newborns. Their excretion rates are directly related to the postnatal age and equalize adult values at 3 or 4 weeks of age. The comparison between preterm infants of gestational age 30 to 33 weeks, showed very similar excretion curves for ampicillin and both present differences with preterm infants with greatergestational age of 34 to 45 weeks [25-26].

PRESCHOOL CHILDREN, SCHOOL CHILDREN AND ADOLESCENTS

Although there are few studies done at these stages of life, most of them indicated that for a variety of medications, children in these ages have an increased metabolic capacity [27].

For instance, drug metabolism was elevated when the half-life elimination of theophylline was determined, a drug that undergoes demethylation through mixed oxidation function. In adolescents, a shorter elimination half-life was obtained than in adults [28].

Likewise, children between 1 and 8 years old metabolize both antipyrine and phenylbutazone much faster than adult individuals. The same phenomenon has been documented for acetaminophen [29].

With regard to the binding of drugs to plasma protein, a lesser variability in the binding of imipramine to plasma proteins was observed in children of 7 to 10 years old, which at puberty gets to the values of an adult. There is virtually no research that evaluated the interaction between active growth and development processes and specific pharmacological principles as well as the influence of disease status.

Immaturity and the general process of growth and development increase the potential risk of intoxication or therapeutic failure and this makes it necessary to have a more substantial knowledge of the problem in such a way that the current approach in which identification of adverse effects is important, should be directed to determine the optimal dose that improves the efficacy and reduce the risk of toxicity. Based on the above, physicians should be aware of the changes in drug doses, which are determined by alterations in drug disposal process at different ages, and also should be aware that adverse drug events can be apparent including many years later [30].

In conclusion, all this goals cannot be achieved without adequate studies of drug disposition in children during the process of growth and development, and who also have pathophysiological disorders such as protein-calorie malnutrition.

REFERENCES

[1] Dost FH. Der Blutspiegel Kinetic Der Konzentrationsabläufe in Der kresilaufflüssigkeit. [Blood levels Kinetic Concentrations in the crescent fluid] *Georg Thieme*, Leipzig, 1953.

[2] Gibaldi M, Perrier D. *Farmacocinetica.* Ed Reverté, S. A. Edición en español, Barcelona España. Reimpresión digital 2006, pp9. [*Pharmacokinetics* Ed Reverté, S. A. Edition in Spanish, Barcelona Spain. Digital Reprint 2006, pp9.]

[3] Wagner JG. *Fundamentals of clinical pharmacokinetics*. Spanish Edition, 1983. Ed Reverte, S. A., Spain: ISBN 84-291-5602-X. pp1-4.

[4] Gibaldi M, Levy G. Pharmacokinetics in clinical practice; 1 concepts *JAMA* 1976;235:1864-7.

[5] Gibaldi M, Perrier D. *Farmacocinetica.* Ed Reverté, S. A. Edición en español, Barcelona España. Reimpresión digital 2006, pp1-45. [*Pharmacokinetics.* Ed Reverté, S. A. Spanish Edition, Barcelona Spain. Digital Reprint 2006, pp1-45].

[6] Gibaldi M, Perrier D. *Farmacocinetica.* Ed Reverté, S. A. Edición en español, Barcelona España. Reimpresión digital 2006, pp45-97. [*Pharmacokinetics.* Ed Reverté, S. A. Edition in Spanish, Barcelona Spain. Digital Reprint 2006, pp1-45.]

[7] Jogiraju VK, Avvari S, Gollen R, Taft DR. Application of physiologically based pharmacokinetic modeling to predict drug disposition in pregnant populations. *Biopharm Drug Dispos* 2017 doi: 10.1002/bdd.2081.

[8] Dean M, Stock B, Patterson RJ, Levy G. Serum protein binding of drugs during and after pregnancy in humans. *Clin Pharmacol Ther* 1980; 28:253-61.

[9] Orueta Sánchez R. López Gil MJ. Manejo de fármacos durante el embarazo. *Inf Ter Sist Nac Salud* 2011;35:107-113. [Management of drugs during pregnancy. *Inf Ter Sist Nac Salud* 2011; 35: 107-113.]

[10] Molina Ortiz D, Camacho Carranza R, Domínguez Ramírez A, Vences Mejía A. Modulación de la expresión de enzimas del citocromo p450 hepáticas durante las etapas fetal y pediátrica. *REB* 2012;31:60-71. [Modulation of the expression of hepatic cytochrome p450 enzymes during the fetal and pediatric stages. *REB* 2012; 31: 60-71.]

[11] Hines RN. Ontogeny of human hepatic cytochromes P450. *J Biochem Mol Toxicol* 2007;21:169-175.

[12] Bartelink I K, Rademaker CMA, Schobben AFAM, Van Den Ander JN: Guidelines on pediatric dosing on the basis of developmental physiology and pharmaco-kinetic considerations. *Clin Pharmacokinet* 2006; 45:1077-97.

[13] Maharaj AR, Edginton AN, Fotaki N. Assessment of age-related changes in pediatric gastrointestinal solubility. *Pharm Res* 2016;33:52-71.

[14] Batchelor HK. Influence of Food on Paediatric Gastrointestinal Drug Absorption Following Oral Administration: A Review. *Children* (Basel) 2015;2:244-71.

[15] Strolin Benedetti M, Baltes EL: Drug metabolism and disposition in children. *Fundam Clin Pharmacol* 2003; 17: 281-99.

[16] Crom WR: Pharmacokinetcis in child. *Environ Health Perspect* 1994;102: 111-18.

[17] Sethi PK, White CA, Cummings BS, Hines RN, Muralidhara S, Bruckner JV. Ontogeny of plasma proteins, albumin and binding of diazepam, cyclosporine, and deltamethrin. *Pediatr Res 2016*;79:409-15.

[18] Matsubara T, Yantada N, Mitomi T, et al.: Cytochrome p-450-dependent monooxygenase activities in prenatal and postnatal human livers: comparison of human liver 7-alkoxycoumarin o-dealkylases with rat liver enzymes. *Jpn J Pharmacol* 1986; 40: 389-98.

[19] Myllynen P, Vähäkangas K. An examination of whether human placental perfusion allows accurate prediction of placental drug transport: studies with diazepam. *J Pharmacol Toxicol Methods* 2002;48:131-8.

[20] Vest MF, Rossier R. Detoxication in the newborn. The ability of the newborn infant to form conjugate with glucuronic acid, glycine, acetate and glutatione. *Ann NY Acad Sci* 1963;111:183-97.

[21] Cavalli R de C, Lanchote VL, Duarte G, Dantas EC, de Prado MF, de Duarte LB. Pharmacokinetics and transplacental transfer of lidocaine and its metabolite for perineal analgesic assistance to pregnant women. *Eur J Clin Pharmacol* 2004;60:569-74.

[22] Sethi PK, White CA, Cummings BS, Hines RN, Muralidhara S, Bruckner JV. Ontogeny of plasma proteins, albumin and binding of diazepam, cyclosporine, and deltamethrin. *Pediatr Res* 2016;79:409-15.

[23] Sereni F, Mandelli M, Principi N, Tognoni G, Pardi G, Morselli PI. Induction of drug metabolizing enzyme activities in the human fetus and in the newborn infant. *Enzyma* 1973;15:318-29.

[24] Juárez-Olguín H, Buendía-Soto E, Lares-Asseff I. Farmacología del feto y el recién nacido. *Gac Med Mex*. 2015; 151: 387-95 [Pharmacology of the fetus and newborn. *Gac Med Mex*. 2015; 151: 387-95.]

[25] Siddiqi A, Khan DA, Khan FA, Razzaq *A. Therapeutic drug monitoring of amikacin in preterm and term infants*. Singapore Med J2009;50:486-9.

[26] Saavedra I, Quiñones L, Saavedra M, Sasso J, León J, Roco A. Farmacocinética de medicamentos de uso pediátrico, visión actual. *Rev Chil Pediatr* 2008;19:249-258 [Pharmacokinetics of medicinal products for pediatric use, current view. *Rev Chil Pediatr* 2008; 19: 249-258.]

[27] Bartelink IK, Rademaker CMA, Schobben AFAM, Van Den Ander JN: Guidelines on pediatric dosing on the basis of developmental physiology and pharmaco-kinetic considerations. *Clin Pharmacokinet* 2006;45:1077-97.

[28] Strolin Benedetti M, Baltes EL. Drug metabolism and disposition in children. *Fundam Clin Pharmacol* 2003; 17:281-99.

[29] Anderson BJ, Woollard GA, Holford NH: A model for size and age changes in the pharmacokinetics of paracetamol in neonates, infants and children. *Br J Clin Pharmacol 2000*;50:125-34.

[30] Kearns GL. Impact of developmental pharmacology on pediatric study design; overcoming the challenges. *J Allergy Clin Immunol* 2000;106:128-39.

In: The Optimization of Drug Prescribing … ISBN: 978-1-53612-263-3
Editor: Hugo Juarez Olguin

Chapter 3

MAIN DISEASES IN PEDIATRICS

Mayra Santillán García*[*]*, Monica Punzo Soto and Belen Juarez Tapia
Laboratorio de Farmacología, Instituto Nacional de Pediatría, Mexico City, Mexico

ABSTRACT

The pediatric age ranges from birth to adolescence and within its chronology, it is divided into periods: newborn, infants, preschool, school, preadolescence and adolescence. During these periods, the child or adolescent must be understood as a subject in development and with constant biological, psychological and social changes, with specific characteristics in each of the stages. The above factors can determine in an important way the health and the onset of diseases. Understanding this is fundamental for any health provider that wants to analyze problems related to childhood. The main causes of illness in patients under 5 years of age are divided into perinatal and postnatal origin. In this chapter, it is intended to address the principal issues leading to postnatal death.

[*] Corresponding Author Email: mayrasant.29@gmail.com

Introduction

At the end of the nineteenth century, 200 of every 1,000 children died before they were a year old, from contagious infectious diseases like dysentery, pneumonia, diphtheria and pertussis [1]. Over the years, it was expected that this tendency would change and that the transmissible diseases would remain in the past as the leading cause of death. Nevertheless, we have witnessed important changes with the passage of the decades and presently in children less than one year old, the main causes of mortality are associated with perinatal problems followed by infectious-contagious diseases. This change has been achieved thanks to preventive programs and strategies, with vaccination having the greatest impact. However, we still have a long way to go in terms of disease prevention.

The pediatric age is divided into periods: newborn, infants, preschool, school, preadolescence and adolescence. During these periods, the child or adolescent must be understood as a subject in development and with constant biological, psychological and social changes, with specific characteristics in each of the stages. The above factors can determine in an important way the health and the onset of diseases. Understanding this is fundamental for any health provider that wants to analyze problems related to childhood. The main causes of illness in patients under 5 years of age are divided into perinatal and postnatal origin. This chapter intends to address the principal issues leading to postnatal death, which are summarized in Figure 1.

Epidemiology

Children under 5 years of age represent 9% of the world population. According to the figures of WHO, 5.9 million children less than five years old died in 2015. On its part, the United Nations International Children´s Emergency Fund (UNICEF) estimates that about 21 children die every minute and more than 80% of these deaths are due to five mostly preventable causes as pneumonia, diarrhea, malaria, neonatal infections and perinatal affectations (Table 1).

It is imperative to bear in mind that many of the children that survive a serious or near-fatal mortal disease will unfortunately not be able to achieve the development of their full potential. Thus, education on and prevention of infectious-contagious diseases are of vital importance.

Table 1. 2015 WHO report on causes of death in children lower than 5 years old

Causes of Death
Pneumonia
Diarrhea
Congenital anomalies
Injuries
Malaria
Measles
HIV/AIDS

Principal Diseases That Affect Pediatric Populations

Pneumonia

Principally, this infection produces affectation of lung parenchyma. The causal agents range from virus and fungi to bacteria. It is the main cause of death in pediatric patients worldwide. In 2015, it led to the death of 920,000 children and only 1/3 of the patients that suffered pneumonia received the correct treatment. Pneumonia is a preventable infection which can be faced with immunization, adequate nutrition and adequate management of environmental factors [2].

Streptococcus Pneumoniae

It is the bacterial agent most frequently associated with community-acquired pneumonia. It is a gram-positive *Diplococcus* and normal member of the respiratory flora. Its virulent factor is owing to the fact that it possesses polysaccharide capsules that can inhibit its phagocytosis. More than 85 different serotypes (antigenic types) capable of provoking pneumonia, otitis media, meningitis and septicemia have been identified [3].

The clinical manifestation swivels on the sudden onset of fever and tachypnea, with a cough appearing after some days. The patients usually adopt a toxic appearance, nevertheless serological and radiological findings can be of great support in clinic diagnosis. The bacteria are not frequently found in blood culture, and are detectable by serological and radiological means in only 4-10% of the cases of community-acquired pneumonia. After the beginning of the application of 7-valent vaccine, a significant reduction in the disease incidence of the vaccinable serotypes has been noticed [4]. The treatment is usually with penicillin, however resistance to this medication and other antibiotics emerges rapidly [3]. The CDC reports a resistance of 2.1% to penicillin and 31.3% to erythromycin. Increased resistance of *S. pneumoniae* to first-line antibiotics has significantly elevated its impact on children´s health. In recent years, *S. pneumoniae* has become increasingly important in countries that vaccinated against *type b H. influenza* due to the falling involvement of this agent in systemic infections, thus placing *S. pneumoniae* as the main etiological agent [5].

Haemophilus Influenzae

It is a gram-negative *coccobacillus* that principally affects children <2 years of age. It is the second most frequent etiologic agent associated with pneumonia worldwide. The most important diseases caused by this infection are pneumonia and meningitis. Vaccination is the only tool capable of preventing the majority of the cases and fortunately it is included in the national program of immunization in more than 90 countries. Efficacy has been reported when administered in early childhood and its application has dramatically reduced the incidence of pneumonia by this agent. Presently, the greatest number of morbidity and mortality cases occurs in developing countries, where vaccination has not been adequately implemented [6].

Diarrhea

This is defined as an increase in the stool numbers or decrease in stool consistency. In these disease, there is an excessive loss of water, electrolytes (sodium, potassium, bicarbonates) and zinc for each evacuation [7].

Table 2. Differential diagnosis of diarrhea in children

Diagnosis	Symptoms
Acute Diarrhea	More than 3 evacuations per day.
	Stool without mucus or blood.
Dysentery	Presence of blood in stool (Reported or seen)
Cholera	Profuse and watery stool, with "rice water color" and severe dehydration data.
	Stool culture positive for Vibrio cholera 01 or 0139
Intestinal intussusception	Blood and mucus in stool.
	Palpable abdominal mass.
	Crying and pallor.
Persistent	Duration ≥14 days

According to WHO, a global mortality from diarrhea among children under 5 years of age is estimated to be 1.87 million, which accounts for 19% of mortality in childhood. Thus, it is considered as the second leading cause of death in infancy, only after pneumonia. 78% of the total death by diarrhea worldwide takes place in Africa and South-East Asia, areas in which the sickness provokes many complications as malnutrition and growth retardation [8]. Both the mortality incidence and risk by diarrheic pathology are greater in children under 1 year of age in whom the most serious threat is dehydration. There are three essential interventions in children with diarrhea: rehydration, zinc supplementation and counseling for continuous feeding [7]. The use of antibiotics is not recommended in children unless there is history of dysentery, suspect of cholera or non-intestinal infections such as urinary tract infection and pneumonia in which the presence of diarrhea is frequent. In Table 2, we summarize the differential diagnosis for any child with diarrhea [7].

Congenital Abnormalities

The congenital abnormalities form the major part of infant morbidity and mortality. Approximately 3% of newborns have a severe or potentially lethal disability [9]. According to WHO 276,000 newborns died each year during the first 5 weeks of life worldwide, from congenital anomalies. The congenital abnormalities are defined as structural and functional abnormalities that occur during intrauterine life and are detected during pregnancy, childbirth or at a later time in life. There are several risk factors associated with congenital alterations (Table 3). The most frequent serious congenital disorders are cardiac malformations, neural tube defects and down syndrome.

Table 3. Risk factors for congenital abnormalities

Risk factors	Conditions
Socioeconomic and demographic factors	Low-income countries (poor diet, exposure to factors that induce or increase the incidence of abnormal perinatal development).
Genetic factors	Advanced maternal age (chromosomal abnormalities), Young mothers (congenital abnomalities).
Infections	Maternal infections such as syphilis or rubella are important cause of congenital abnormalities.
Nutritional status of the mother	Iodine and folates deficiency, overweight and diseases such as diabetes mellitus are related with some congenital abnormalities. In addition, excessive vitamin A intake may affect the normal development of the embryo or fetus.
Environmental factors	Maternal exposure to certain pesticides and other chemical products.

Congenital Heart Diseases

Congenital heart diseases are the most common malformations. Its incidence is 5-12 per 1,000 live births. Congenital heart disease is defined as any structural abnormality of the heart or the great vessels. They are the result of alterations in the third and tenth week of gestation [10]. Congenital heart diseases that present a greater possibility of prenatal diagnosis are the most severe ones due to alterations of the 4 chambers or outflow tracts and are considered to be associated with increased risk of neonatal death. They are frequently related to chromosomal defects and other extra-cardiac malformations reason why it is difficult to demonstrate an advantage from prenatal diagnosis of congenital heart diseases [11]. The most common congenital heart diseases are divided into 2 groups:

Cyanotic Congenital Heart Diseases

Based on their pathophysiology, they are subdivided into reduced and increased blood flow.

Reduced Blood Flow

This includes:

- Tetralogy of Fallot
- Pulmonary atresia
- Tricuspid atresia
- Total anomalous pulmonary venous drainage

Increased Blood Flow

This includes:

- Transposition of the great vessels.
- Single ventricle

- Arterial trunk
- Some forms of total anomalous pulmonary venous drainage

Acyanotic Congenital Heart Diseases

These include:

- Interventricular communication (IVC)
- Interauricular communication (IAC)
- Persistent arterial duct (PAD)
- Aortic stenosis
- Pulmonary stenosis
- Coarctation of the Aorta
- Atrioventricular canal (defect of endocardial relief)

Table 4 shows the most common congenital heart diseases [12-16].

Neural Tube Defects

These defects constitute most of the congenital abnormalities of the central nervous system (CNS) and derive from the failure of the spontaneous closure of the neural tube between the third and fourth week of intrauterine development [17] (Table 5, [18, 19]).

Down Syndrome

Down syndrome (DS) forms part of the most important cause of intellectual disabilities. It is associated with different congenital pathologies among which are heart diseases, leukemia, Alzheimer, Hirschsprung etc.

Table 4. The most common congenital heart diseases

Heart diseases	Definition	Prevalence	Clinical Picture	Diagnosis	Treatment
Tetralogy of Fallot	It is a heart disease of the conotruncal family. The major defect is the previous deviation of the infundibular septum formed by: Pulmonary stenosis Interventricular Communication Aortic cavalry Right ventricular Hypertrofy	10% of the congenital heart diseases	If pulmonary obstruction is severe and pulmonary flow is reduced, cyanosis occurs. Paroxystic hypercyanotic attack (1st and 2nd year of life). Dyspnea of effort. Moderate obstruction. Balanced systemic and pulmonary flow. Systolic murmur in superior parasternal border. Severe obstruction, hypoxic crisis, the murmur disappears, left-right flow.	Electrocardiogram Chest Radiography, Doppler echocardiography, Cardiac Catheterization	Severe cyanosis. PGE1 to maintain ductus open and Subsequent surgery. Hypoxic crisis. Morphine IV and bolus of liquid. B-Blockers (propranolol), and surgery.
Interventricular Communication	The defects are located in any area of the interventricular septum but majority are membranous type.	Common Malformation. 25% of all the congenital heart diseases.	Congestive heart failure may appear between 2 to 3 weeks of life with galloping rhythm, tachycardia, tachypnea drainage, hepatomegaly, poor peripheral perfusion, systolic murmur.	Electrocardiogram Chest X-ray, Echocardiogram-Doppler	Medical treatment will be indicated for infants with clinical cardiac failure and delay in stature. 1. Diuretics 2. Angiotensin converting enzyme inhibitors (ACAI). 3. Digoxin. Adequate prophylaxis for respiratory infections.

Table 4. (Continued)

Heart diseases	Definition	Prevalence	Clinical Picture	Diagnosis	Treatment
Interauricular Communication.	Opening in the Interauricular septum. It is classified based on its position in relation to oval fosa, embryogenesis and size: CIA ostium secundum type CIA of the venous sinus CIA of the coronary sinus CIA ostiumprimum	10-15% often appears in isolation in adolescents and adults.	Right ventricular overload: Increased right ventricular impulse. Soft ejection systolic murmur at the left sternal border with extended, fixed and unfolded second cardiac noise. Diastolic protomesic murmur.	Chest X-ray Electrocardiogram Echocardiogram Cardiac catheterization	Closing communication is indicated when there is significant short-circuit. Elective closing age is from 3 to 5 years old. *
Aortic Coarctation	It is a congenital heart disease manifested as stenosis of the aortic arc. Majority occurs near the ductus arteriosus.	6-8%	The symptom depends on the age of presentation and degree of obstruction. Peripheral pulses are diminished in lower limbs. Presence of systolic murmur in the left sternal border that is transmitted to the back and neck.	Confirmative diagnosis. Echocardiogram. Angiography	Surgery is the treatment of election.
Persistent arteriosus Duct	It is a vascular structure that connects the proximal descending aorta the main pulmonary artery near the origin of the left pulmonary branch. It is essential during feta life. It closes spontaneously after birth.	The incidence varies from 20% in preterm infants >32 weeks of gestation to 60% in preterm infants of <28 weeks of gestation.	Clinical pictures comprise of systolic injection murmur with less continuous frequency. It is better auscultated in left infraclavicular region and left superior parasternal with irradiation to the back. Hyperdynamic pericardium, tachycardia, bulging pulses in postductal region, polypnea, apnea and hepatomegaly.	Clinic Echocardiogram	The treatment in newborns is a controversial topic.

Taken from (Apitz 2009, [12]), (Spicer 2014, [13]), (Adiele 2014, [14]), (Torok 2015, [15]), (Abdel-Hady 2013, [16]).

Table 5. Characteristics of the main types ofneural tube defects (NTDs)

	Anencephaly	**Myelomeningocele (open spina bifida; SB)**	**Craniorachischisis**	**Spinal dysraphism**	**Encephalocele**
Relative frequency	40%	50%	3%	Unknown	7%
Epidemiological features	Typical of NTDs as a whole; mostly sporadic	Typical of NTDs as a whole; mostly sporadic	Unknown; high prevalence noted in North China	Unknown	Usually sporadic, but can be syndromic (e.g., in Meckel syndrome)
Sex ratio (F:M)	Marked female excess (3:1)	Variable in different populations; approximately equal overall	Female excess, as for anencephaly	Equal	Female excess among occipital lesions
Clinical presentation	Lack of brain and cranial vault; fetal loss or stillbirth	Open spinal cord covered by meningeal sac (SB cystic) or exposed (SB open); most commonly thoraco-lumbar, lumbar or lumbo-sacral; usually live birth; frequently associated with hydrocephalus post-natally	Anencephaly continuous with complete open spina bifida; fetal loss or stillbirth	Skin covered lesion involving 2 or more vertebrae, apparent only on radiography; hair tuft, lipoma or another cutaneous feature often co-exists	Meningeal sac, often containing brain tissue, protrudes from skull; commonly in occipital, parietal or fronto-ethmoidal locations
Prenatal diagnosis	Ultrasound from first trimester; elevated serum AFP	Ultrasound from first trimester; elevated serum AFP	Ultrasound from first trimester; elevated serum AFP	No	Ultrasound, depending on size of lesion
Surgical treatment	None: lethal beyond birth	Surgical closure post-natally or *in utero* in some centres; insertion of cerebro-spinal fluid shunt for hydrocephalus	None: lethal beyond birth	Untethering of spinal cord, usually in childhood	Repair by removal of sac and closure

Table 5. (Continued)

	Anencephaly	Myelomeningocele (open spina bifida; SB)	Craniorachischisis	Spinal dysraphism	Encephalocele
Genetic causation	Genes as for NTDs as a whole (see text)	Genes as for NTDs as a whole (see text)	Planar cell polarity genes are only positive findings	Unknown	*MKS1-3, RPGRIP1L, CEP290* genes all identified as causal for Meckel syndrome (occipital encephalocele)
Non-genetic causation	Increased risk in diabetic pregnancy; no specific associations	Valproic acid exposure increases risk 10X; increased risk in diabetic pregnancy	None known	None known	None known
Primary prevention	FA, as for NTDs as a whole	FA, as for NTDs as a whole; inositol prevention of open spinal bifida in *Grhl3* mouse model	FA may prevent: North China frequency declined after FA introduced	FA-resistant? Lipomyelomeningocele frequency shows no decline after food fortification with FA	FA may prevent: some evidence of decline after food fortification with FA
Embryonic origin	Failure of cranial neural tube closure	Failure of caudal neuropore closure	Failure of Closure 1	Defective secondary neurulation	Post-neurulation disorder?
Pathogenesis	Originates after failed closure as exencephaly; converted to anencephaly by degeneration of neural tissue and absence of cranial vault formation	Degeneration of exposed neural tissue following failed closure; origin of meningeal sac in SB cystic is not clear	Combined anencephaly and myelomeningocele	Unknown	Herniation of meninges with or without brain tissue through defect in skull

*Relative frequencies relate to NTDs in established pregnancies. Based on data taken from: (Dolk 1991, [18]), (Johnson 2004, [19]).

The incidence of trisomy 21 is influenced by maternal age and differs from the population between 1 in 319 and 1 in 1000 newborns [20]. In developed countries, the average life expectancy for DS is 55 years [21]. In 95% of cases, DS is caused by trisomy of the chromosome 21 due to meiotic disjunction in the ovule. Other causes can be Robertsionan translocation and the isochromosomal chromosome or mosaicism [22]. DS can be diagnosed during pregnancy through cytogenetic study of chorionic villi or amniotic liquid or by ultrasound in the first trimester of pregnancy. In the second trimester, this can be done by biochemical study in search of four biochemical markers alpha-fetoprotein, total HCCG, unconjugated estradiol and free β-hCG. In the first trimester, the screening can also be done using a combination of nuchal transluscency ultrasound and β-hCG-free maternal serum biochemical markers and pregnancy-associated plasma protein-A (PAPP-A) [23].

The importance of timely diagnosis of DS at prenatal and birth lies on preventing the morbidity and mortality in this type of patients. In a study carried out by Castro [24], a follow-up of patients with diagnosis of DS was made during the first years of life with the observation that the causes of death in the patients were associated to digestive and congenital heart diseases. Fewer complications due to in-hospital infections were reported. Adequate follow-up and diagnosis of these patients would improve their prognosis and quality of life.

ACCIDENTS

According to the report of WHO, more than 2000 children die each day from unintentional (accidental) injuries, and each year tens of millions of children are admitted in hospitals for injuries that often leave them disabled for life. The five principal causes of death due to injuries are:

1. Motor vehicle accidents with a toll of 260,000 deaths in children and about ten million injuries. Motor vehicle accidents are the

main cause of death in the group of 10 to 19 years of age and one of the principal causes of disability in children.

2. Drowning has a toll of 175,000 deaths in children per year and about 3 million cases of children who survived incidents of such accident. The brain lesion which drowning leaves in some survivors makes non-fatal drowning the type of accident with the greatest health and economic impact in the life of victims.
3. Fire-burns register a toll of 96,000 deaths in children per year. Its mortality rate is 11 times greater in low- and middle-income countries than in high-income ones.
4. Falls have a toll of 47,000 deaths in children and hundreds of thousands of non-fatal injuries in this group of people.
5. Unintentional poisoning leaves a toll of 45,000 deaths in children per year [25].

More than 90% of deaths by accidents occur in low- and middle-income countries where preventive measures are not implemented and whose health system are less prepared to cope with such incidents [26].

It is important to know the main causes of death by accidents in order to implement preventive measures aimed at reducing mortality rate and number of sequels by accidents. Each country must prepare their health professionals to provide better care to victims of accident and implement programs aimed towards its prevention.

Malaria

Malaria is a re-emergent infection of parasitic origin, which in spite of the great international efforts to eradicate it, continues to have a significant prevalence with a report in 2015 of 214 million cases of which 292,000 were children. The disease causes 306,000 deaths in children lower than 5 years of age at a world wide level. The infection occurs mainly in developing countries and it is one of the principal infectious causes of death only after respiratory and gastrointestinal infections [27].

It is an infection caused by a parasite belonging to the genus Plasmodium. To date, 5 species - Plasmodium falciparum, P. vivax, P. ovale, P. malariae and P. knowlesi - responsible for the disease have been identified in humans, with P. falciparum being the most prevalent in Africa and East Asian countries, regions in which the disease is highly prevalent [28].

The life cycle of the parasite involves two hosts, Anopheles mosquito and the human. When malaria infected mosquito bites the human, it inoculates the sporozoites which initiate a pre-erythrocytic phase and then pass to the asexual erythrocytic phase, a stage in which the symptoms that lead to the disease and its complications appear. At this stage, parasitemia occurs and if a mosquito of the genus Anopheles bites the infected person again, the mosquito is infected and the multiplication of the parasite begins again. The developed parasites are deposited in the salivary gland of the mosquito where it stays until the mosquito bites a new human host to infect him.

The disease mainly affects children with a maximum incidence between 2 and 10 years. In a non-immunized person, the incubation period is from 6 to 14 days. The pre-latent stage which ranges from the inoculation of the sporozoite to parasitemia is 10 days. The symptoms appear between 7 and 15 days after the mosquito bite. Clinically, the disease is characterized by unspecific symptomatology such as fever, headache, myalgia, cough, vomiting, diarrhea and abdominal pain.

The disease can be treated in only 48 hours; however, it is capable of provoking fatal complications if the diagnosis and treatment are delayed or if there is a short and long term relapse or a “recrudescence”.

Treatment for malaria should ideally start within the first 24 hours of the onset of the symptoms, otherwise it may progress to a serious illness that can lead to death. On the other hand, if the patient does not continue the treatment, clinical relapses can occur weeks or months after the first infection. These relapses may occur even after 60 days in case of infection by P. vivax and P. ovale. Such relapse is due to the reactivation of the hypnozoites that are still present in the liver. In the case of P. falciparum and P. malaria, if the treatment is discontinued, the patient presents "recrudescence" which is due to the survival of the parasite in the erythrocytes [28].

To date, there are 4 groups of antimalarial drugs which are directed to attacking the asexual phase of the infection (erythrocytic phase) which is symptomatic. In spite of having a directed drug, none of them is capable of eliminating all the strains of the parasite, thus, the reason why one or more combinations are frequently used. The choice of the combination depends on both the local incidence of the parasite and severity of the presentation. The most commonly used combination is a combined therapy with artemisinin (CTA). Presently, resistance to some antimalarial drugs mainly chloroquine has been reported, however resistance to other drugs as mefloquine, halofantrine and artemisinin has also been reported [29].

For its prevention, WHO proposes a global strategy against malaria 2016-2030 with the objective of reducing the mortality to 90% in comparison with 2015. Because it is a vector-borne disease, the main preventive measure is to avoid being bitten by a mosquito of the genus Anopheles. Thus, in countries with high incidence, it is recommended to sleep under Insecticide-Treated Bed Net (ITBN). On the other hand, starting from 2014 the *Strategic Advisory Group of Experts* (SAGE) and the *Malaria Policy Advisory Committee* (MPAC) recommended the pilot implementation of the first malaria vaccine (RTS, S/ASO1). However, it is not yet recommended at a worldwide level [27, 30].

MEASLES

It is a common contagious exanthematic disease which in spite of available safe and efficacious vaccine for its prevention, continued to constitute one of the principal childhood pathogens worldwide with a toll of 130,000 deaths in 2015 at world level [31]. The disease is caused by a virus of the measles that belong to the genus Morbillivirus from the family of Paramixoviridae [32]. It is part of the family of the etiological agents for diseases as parotiditis. These viruses share the same genomic structural characteristics for having a simple single-stranded RNA molecule and negative polarity. Measles virus is a neurotrophic virus that is capable of invading the central nervous system, causing encephalitis and peripheral nerve infections and deafness. Infection by measles is the principal cause of infectious deafness in the world and also has a high incidence of causing blindness. The first manifestation is fever which is usually seen 10-12 days after exposition to the virus and lasts between 4 and 7 days. In the initial phase, the patient can present rhinorrhea, cough, coryza as well as Koplic classic sign characterized by the presence of whitish macules in the inner portion of the cheeks near the third molar. Subsequent, there appears exanthemas first on the scalp and retroauricular, and then extends to caudal cephalus, from where it spreads to reach the hands and legs in two or three days. The exanthema usually last for 5 to 6 days and disappears. The interval between the exposition to the virus and appearance of exanthema is 7 to 18 days (average 14 days). As mentioned above, the main cause of death in children lower than 5 years due to measles infection are secondary to their complications and 41% of them have some complications. Among the most frequent are acute otitis media (14%), diarrhea (11.5%), pneumonia (8.6%), encephalitis (0.2%), blindness and deafness. These complications are more frequent and potentially fetal in malnourished or immuno-deficient children such as HIV/AIDS infection [31].

Patients may also present late complications such as inclusion body encephalitis (MIBE), which emerges as an immune response against the virus of measles leading to myeloencephalitis post-measles with a high degree of mortality and manifested months after infection in immune compromised patients. This encephalitis presents a progressive course and after some months of evolution causes death. Measles has been the first persistent viral infection associated with the central nervous system. Years or decades after the infection, the majority of the patients who had the infection in the first two years of life may present Subacute Sclerosing Panencephalitis (SSPE). This disease or complication has a progressive course of years to even decades. Cell death by apoptosis of neurons and glia cells including oligodendrocytes has been observed and in an advanced stage, demyelination and brain atrophy, until it causes the death of the patient [33].

So far there is no specific antiviral agent against the treatment of measles virus. However, supportive treatment should be provided for any complications presented by the patient to ensure adequate nutrition, hydration or replacement of fluids or electrolytes in children with some degree of dehydration secondary to vomiting and diarrhea. The use of antibiotics is exclusively indicated for patients that presented co-infection as pneumonia, otitis or bacterial conjunctivitis. In addition to supportive treatment, all children diagnosed of measles should receive vitamin A supplementation regardless of their nutritional status. This supplementation, according to some studies, could support the prevention of blindness and other eye injuries as well as the reduction of mortality by up to 50%.

As to prevention, vaccination against measles virus has been in use for more than 50 years and it is considered safe, efficacious and accessible for the world economy. Vaccination has provided a great benefit by reducing global mortality. The vaccine is usually combined with rubella and/or parotiditis vaccines applied during the immunization campaign in countries that report a high incidence and mortality. The report of WHO shows that in 2015, 85% of the world´s children population received a dose of the vaccine before one year of life. Nevertheless, approximately 15% of the children do not achieve immunity with the first dose, so to guarantee immunity and prevent possible outbreaks, it is recommended to apply two doses [34].

HIV

The human immunodeficiency virus disease is presently a devastating sickness that affects both the physical health and survival of thousands of children, and destroys families depriving them of love, attention and protection. Mother-to-child transmission of HIV contributes significantly to the transmission of the virus. At the advent of the disease, it was estimated 260,000 children were affected by HIV and by 2012, 3.3 million children have been infected [35]. The transmission of HIV occurs when a seropositive woman transmits the virus to her baby during pregnancy, labor and delivery or postpartum through breastfeeding. If they do not receive prophylactic treatment, 15-30% of the infants born to seropositive women will be infected by HIV during pregnancy or childbirth and 5-15% will be infected on being breastfed [36].

WHO has been in charge of carrying out minimum goals with high impact on mother-to-child transmission. The goals are to have less than 50 infantile infections per 100,000 live births and transmission rate of less than 5% in the population groups that practice breastfeeding and less than 2% in the groups that do not practice it. To achieve these objectives, the following goals must be met:

1) Coverage of prenatal care to the tune of or greater than 95%.
2) Coverage of HIV detection tests.
3) Coverage of antiretroviral treatment for HIV-positive pregnant women equal or greater than 90%.

Adult patients with HIV share common characteristics with afflicted children such as immunosuppression caused by the destruction of CD4+ lymphocytes as well as the direct and indirect pathogenic effects on other organs. The latter is more relevant in the newborn and infants for coinciding with the phases of ontogenesis and differentiation [37]. The risk of developing AIDS is greater in children than in adults and it is especially high in the first year of life (20-30%). This tendency decreases each year by 2-3% starting from the first year. There is a greater increase in the risk of progressing to AIDS or death at 12 months when CD4 is below 15-20%. For this, the CD4 lymphocyte count is used for antiretroviral treatment decisions.

Depending on the pharmacotherapy chosen, the pharmacokinetic parameters of pediatric patients may differ from the adult due to the continuous growth and maturation of the organs involved in the metabolism and elimination of drugs. Initiation of treatment aims to maximally suppress viral replication. The cost-benefit of the treatment should always be assessed and parents should be sensitized on the highest possible adherence to the treatment, because this is related tovirological and clinical response [38].

Early maternal and infant diagnosis and the immediate commencement of antiretroviral treatment should be part of the most important approach. That is why the most important goal is to prevent the newborn from being infected.

REFERENCES

[1] Tschudy MM, Arcara KM. (Eds.) (2012). *The Harriet Lanehand book: A manual for pediatric house officers*. Philadelphia, PA: Mosby Elsevier.

[2] Integrated Management of ChildhoodIllness (IMCI). *WHO recommendations on the management of diarrhoea and pneumonia in HIV-infected infants and children.* Geneva: World Health Organization; 2010.

[3] Patterson MJ. Chapter 13 Streptococcus; In: Baron S, editor. *Medical Microbiology.* 4th edition. Galveston TX: University of Texas Medical Branch at Galveston; 1996.

[4] Méndez-Lage S, Losada-Castillo I, Agulla-Budiño A. Streptococcus pneumoniae: Serotype distribution, antimicrobial susceptibility, risk factors and mortality in Galicia over a two year-period. *Enferm Infecc Microbiol Clin* 2015; 33:579-84.

[5] *Centers for Disease Control and Prevention Active Bacterial Core Surveillance Report*, Emerging Infections Program Network, (2010)

[6] Watt JP, Wolfson LJ, O'Brien KL, Henkle E, Deloria-Knoll M, McCall N, Lee E, Levine OS, Hajjeh R, Mulholland K, Cherian T; Hib and Pneumococcal Global Burden of Disease Study Team. Burden of disease caused by Haemophilus influenzae type b in children younger than 5 years: global estimates. *Lancet* 2009; 374:903-11

[7] *Pocket book of hospital care for children: Guidelines for the management of common childhood illnesses* – 2nd ed. 2013.

[8] Boschi-Pinto C, Velebit L, Shibuyac K. Estimating child mortality due to diarrhea in developing countries. *Bull World Health Organ* 2008; 86: 710–717.

[9] Lowry RB. Common Congenital Anomalies. *Can Fam Phys* 1985; 31:1033–1037.

[10] Perich C. Cardiopatías congénitas más frecuentes. *Pediatr integral* 2008; 12:807-818.

[11] Yates R. The influence of prenatal diagnosis on outcome in patients with structural congenital heart disease. *Prenatal Diagn* 2004; 24:1143-9.

[12] Apitz C, Webb GD. Tetralogy of Fallot. *Lancet.* 2009; 374:1462-71.

[13] Spicer D E, Hsu HH, Co-Vu J, Anderson RH, Fricker FJ. Ventricular septal defect. *Orphanet J. Rare Dis* 2014;9: 144.

[14] Adiele DK, Chinawa JM, Arodiwe IO, Gouthami V, Murthy KS, Eze JC, Obidike EO, Ujunwa FA. Atrial septal defects: Pattern, clinical profile, surgical techniques and outcome at Innova heart hospital: A 4-year review. *Nigerian Med J* 2014; 55:126-129.

[15] Torok RD, Campbell MJ, Fleming GA, Hill KD. Coarctation of the aorta: Management from infancy to adulthood. *World J Cardiol* 2015; 7,765-775.

[16] Abdel-Hady H, Nasef N, Shabaan AE, Nour I. Patent Ductus Arteriosus in Preterm Infants: Do We Have the Right Answers? *Bio Med Res Int* 2013, 676192.

[17] Greene N, Copp A. Neural tube Defects. *Annu Rev Neurosci* 2014; 37:221-42.

[18] Dolk H, De Wals P, Gillerot Y, Lechat MF, Ayme S, Cornel M, Cuschieri A, Garne E, Goujard J, Laurence KM, Heterogeneity of neural tube defects in Europe: The significance of site of defect and presence of other major anomalies in relation to geographic differences in prevalence. *Teratology* 1991; 44:547-59.

[19] Johnson KMK, Suarez L, Felkner MM, Hendricks K. Prevalence of craniorachischisis in a Texas-Mexico border population. Birth Defects Res Part A. *Clin Mol Teratol* 2004 70:92-4.

[20] Wahab AA, Bener A, Teebi AS. The incidence patterns of Down syndrome in Qatar. *Clin Genet* 2006; 69:360-2.

[21] Glasson EJ, Sullivan SG, Hussain R, Petterson BA, Montgomery PD, Bittles AH. The changing survival profile of people with Down's syndrome: implications for genetic counselling. *Clin Genet* 2002; 62:390-3.

[22] Epstein CJ, Scriver CR, Beaudet AL, Sly WS, Valle D, editors. *The Metabolic & Molecular Bases of Inherited Disease.* New York: McGraw-Hill; 2001. pp. 1223–1256.

[23] Spencer K. Screening for Down syndrome. *Scand J Clin Lab Invest Suppl* 2014; 244:41-7.

[24] Castro Al. Mortalidad y enfermedades asociadas al síndrome de Down en el primer año de vida, *Arch Pediatr Urug* 2007; 78:3. [Castro Al. Mortality and diseases associated with Down syndrome in the first year of life, *Arch Pediatr Urug* 2007; 78:3.]

[25] Peden M, Oyegbite K, Ozanne-Smith J, Hyder AA, Branche C, Rahman AKMF, Rivara F, Bartolomeos K, editors. World Report on *Child Injury Prevention.* Geneva: World Health Organization; 2008.

[26] Goseelin S. Los traumatismos. El problema sanitario desatendido en los países de desarrollo. Boletin de la Organización Mundial de Salud 2009; 87:245-324. [Goseelin S. Trauma. The neglected health problem in developing countries. *WHO* 2009; 87:245-324.]

[27] *World Malaria Report 2016*. Geneva: World Health Organization; 2016.

[28] Douglas NM, Pontororing GJ, Lampah DA, Yeo TW, Kenangalem E, Poespoprodjo JR et al. Mortality attributable to Plasmodium vivax malaria: a clinical audit from Papua, Indonesia. *BMC Med* 2014; 12:217.

[29] WHO Global Technical Strategy for Malaria 2016– 2030. Geneva: World Health Organization (WHO); 2015 (Roll Back Malaria Partnership. Action and investment to defeat malaria 2016–2030. *For a Malaria free World.* Geneva.

[30] *WHO*. 2015. (http://www.rollbackmalaria.org/files/files/aim/RBM_AIM_Report_A4_EN-Sept2015.pdf, accessed 16 November 2016).

[31] Cibulskis RE, Aregawi M, Williams R, Otten M, Dye C. Worldwide incidence of malaria in 2009: Estimates, time trends, and a critique of methods. *PLoS Med* 2011;8: e1001142.

[32] WHO. *Global Measles and Rubella Strategic Plan* 2012-2020 [Internet]. Ginebra (Suiza): OMS; 2012.

[33] Griffin DE. Measles Virus. In: Fields BN, Knipe DM, Howley PM, editors. *Fields Virology*. Philadelphia: Lippincott-Raven Publishers, 2007; pp 1551-85.

[34] O'Hagan DT. Recent developments in vaccine delivery system. In: Levine M, Koper JB, Rappuoli R, Liu MA, Good MF, editors. *New generation vaccines*. 3a ed. Nueva York: Marcel Dekker, 2004. pp 259-70.

[35] WHO. Global Vaccine Action Plan. Monitoring Evaluation and Accountability. *Secretariat Annual Report 2016* [Internet]. Ginebra (Suiza): OMS; 2016.

[36] *Report on the Global AIDS Epidemic*. Ginebra, ONUSIDA. 2013.

[37] De Cock KM, Fowler MG, Mercier E, de Vincenzi I, Saba J, Hoff E, Alnwick DJ, Rogers M, Shaffer N. Prevention of mother-to-child HIV transmission in resource-poor countries: translating research into policy and practice. *JAMA* 2000; 283:1175-82.

[38] Gatell JM, Clotet B, Podzamczer D, Practical Guide of AIDS. *Clinic, diagnosis and treatment*. 7ª edition.

[39] Guidelines for the Use of Antiretroviral Agents in Pediatric HIV Infection. *DHHS*. November 2004.

In: The Optimization of Drug Prescribing … ISBN: 978-1-53612-263-3
Editor: Hugo Juarez Olguin © 2018 Nova Science Publishers, Inc.

Chapter 4

How Is the LADME Process of Drugs in Children?

***Hugo Juarez Olguín*[1,2,*]*, David Calderón Guzmán*[3] *and Mónica Punzo Soto*[1,2]**

[1]Laboratorio de Farmacología, Instituto Nacional de Pediatría, Mexico City, Mexico

[2]Departamento de Farmacología, Facultad de Medicina, Universidad Nacional Autónoma de Mexico. Mexico

[3]Laboratorio de Neurociencias, Instituto Nacional de Pediatría, Mexico City, Mexico

Abstract

LADME refers to the biological pathway which the drugs follow after administration. Such pathway comprises of five processes: liberation, absorption, distribution, metabolism and excretion. Each of the processes is closely related with the therapeutic and toxic effects of a drug. Hence, it is extremely important to take into account the way a drug is administered as well as its pharmaceutical presentation. While most of

* Corresponding Author Email: juarezol@yahoo.com

the references on the study of the pathway have been on adult; in children, the studies performed so far has been very little. Nevertheless, the studies on the topic have recently increased for being considered a crucial area of risk. The present chapter takes a deeper look at the pattern of the profile of LADME process in children.

INTRODUCTION

An important branch of pharmacology is the study of the pathway of drugs in time course and dose through an organism. Such pathway encompasses the processes of liberation, absorption, distribution, metabolism and elimination of drugs designated as LADME route.

In the debut of '70s of XX century, the WHO defined pharmacokinetic as the study of liberation, absorption, distribution, metabolism and elimination of drugs [1].

The acronym LADME was adopted to facilitate the comprehension of these parameters.

- **Liberation**: release of drug from the pharmaceutical form.
- **Absorption**: access of the unaltered drug into the blood circulation.
- **Distribution**: the transportation of drug to different parts of the body.
- **Metabolism**: biotransformation of the original molecule to one or various metabolites that are less toxic and efficacious than the unaltered form (unmetabolized form).
- **Elimination**: excretion of the drug or the metabolites from the body via different routes (renal, biliary, salivary, etc.) [2].

Some authors consider the process of liberation as a part of this pathway for the fact that it implies a series of engineering and technical knowledge inherent in the elaboration and stability of the pharmaceutical forms, which are important for the release of the active ingredient or drug from their excipients and hence may affect, to a large extent, the absorption

[3]. For a drug to exert its action after being released, it needs to be absorbed, transported to the appropriate tissues or organs, penetrate into the corresponding subcellular structure and induce a response or alteration in the ongoing process of the structure. The drug could be distributed in the simultaneous or sequential form in different tissues, get fixed or stored, be metabolized to yield active and inactive metabolites and finally be eliminated. Each of the processes is closely related with the therapeutic and toxic effects of a drug hence, it is paramount to take into account not only the form of administration but also the type of pharmaceutical presentation of a drug. During the processes of absorption, distribution, biotransformation and elimination, the drug must pass through some biological membranes.

How Is LADME Process in Children?

There have been little studies in the process of drug release in children. It is frequent to find the administration of solid drugs such as tablets, capsules or pills in the early stages of a child´s life. Nevertheless, when it is decided to use them, their characteristics like disintegration and dissolution time of the tablets ought to be considered since they constitute an indispensable requisite for the onset of absorption. A special case is the suppositories, where the mechanisms of the liberation of the active substance in the anorectal zone and its adequate availability are well established. Once a drug is absorbed and passed into the vascular system, it begins to circulate either in free form or bond to blood proteins and be distributed throughout the body where the manifestation of its effects takes place. The drug is then eliminated via hepatic biotransformation in conjunction with renal excretion. Based on this, it is pertinent that pediatricians have precise knowledge of the physiopathology of the common problems in children for proper therapeutic intervention. The age of a child, the height and body weight are the variables to consider since the pharmacological activity of a drug depends on such variables and are in close relationship with the first years of life. In infants, the principal factor responsible for the variability in the action of drugs is the age.

Hypersensitivity to drugs is common in children. Their response is located on the extreme left of the dose-response and normal distribution curves. It is believed that this increase in hypersensitivity is due to modifications in the pharmacokinetic processes of liberation, absorption, distribution, metabolism and excretion [4].

The Newborn

Birth is usually accompanied by a series of anatomical and physiological changes in the newborn, which are necessary for his or her adaptation to the new external environment [5]. For this, the management of drugs by the body in this stage is different from what occurs in later stages of life. It is evident that morphological and physiological changes, modify the absorption of drugs. In birth, some modifications as bacterial colonization and rapid alterations in splenic circulation take place. The available surface area influences the speed and magnitude of absorption and it is different in older ages, the gastrointestinal tract is the portion of the body with the biggest surface area in the newborn [6].

It seems that at early ages, there is increased activity in the intestinal permeability and this permits easier passage of molecules. The gastrointestinal absorption of drugs is subject to two controlling factors: pH-dependent diffusion and the gastric emptying time that undergo continuous changes after birth [7]. At birth, the gastric pH is within the limits of neutrality (6.0 – 8.0) which descends to the range of 1.0 – 3.0 in the first 24 hours and becomes relatively achlorhydric in the next nine days. At three years of age, gastric pH values attain the status of adult pH values. The low gastric acidity explains the low concentrations of some penicillin in newborns when compared with older kids [8]. Gastric emptying time also varies with age. It is usually lower in newborn in relation to adults, a situation that remains until six months of age, even when intestinal movements are irregular and unpredictable and could be changed by diet and feeding schedules [9]. In intramuscular or subcutaneous administration of drugs, the absorption speed depends on the regional blood flow, which changes during the first two weeks of life. There are variations in blood flow in different muscle groups and this can be higher under hypoxic conditions [10].

ABSORPTION

The access of a drug to the site of action requires first its passage to the circulatory system. This movement of a drug primarily depends on the passage of the active substance through the tissue cell membranes involved. The absorption of a drug, after oral administration, is influenced by its specific characteristics such as the speed of dissolution, solubility in water and the degree of ionization. Due to age related changes, it is pertinent to consider the host and his or her peculiarities. For instance, absorption is modified by the gastrointestinal content, the pH, intestinal motility, gastric emptying time and mesenteric blood flow among others [11].

The absorption speed will affect the time and duration of maximum concentration, but not the area under the concentration curve in function of time. Gastrointestinal absorption is affected by changes in maturation that takes place right from birth due to changes in the gastric secretion volume, intestinal motility and blood flow. Gastric emptying is directly affected by different factors (Table 1). Moreover, food composition influences in the absorption velocity since gastric emptying time depends on food density and the type of fatty acid it contains. Hence, the absorption of drugs which takes place in the stomach could be faster than expected when the speed of gastric emptying is altered. Some authors have observed that human milk stimulates gastric emptying more than milk formula. Drugs with high affinity for proteins or those that are liposoluble may not rapidly be absorbed by the stomach when a child receives formula because of the continuous presence of milk in the stomach. The poor absorption of some weak bases as methylxanthines in advanced ages mainly due to low pH, do not occur in newborns for having reduced gastric acid secretion and high pH [12]. When these limitations are not considered in the calculation of drug doses in the newborn, toxic effects are produced (Table 2).

Table 1. Factors that influence in gastric emptying speed in newborns

Decreases gastric emptying speed	Increases gastric emptying speed
- Premature	- Maternal milk
- Gastroesophageal reflux	- Hypocaloric food
- Respiratory stress syndrome	
- Cardiac diseases	
- Long chain fatty acid	

Table 2. Factors affecting oral absorption of drugs in newborns

Factors	Differences in the newborn	Effect on drug absorption
pH	High	Affects nonionic diffusion and chemical stability of drugs.
Small intestinal pH	High	Variable: may change metabolism models
Microbial flora	Decreased and qualitatively different	May decrease the total amount: could cause a greater variation in amount and speed
Peristalsis	Irregular	Decreases absorption speed of drugs absorbed in the duodenum
Gastric emptying time	Slow	

The absorption of most drugs takes place in the small intestine with a bigger area of absorption and specialized cells for this assignment. The type of bacteria and the level of its colonization influence in the absorption of some drugs. If the fetal intestine is virtually sterile, there is a rapid colonization of bacteria at birth based on the type of food given to the baby.

In the neonatal stage, on one part, the bacterial flora plays an important role in the hydrolysis of conjugated drugs secreted in the bile while on the other part, intestinal bacteria could affect the absorption of certain vitamins like K vitamin. Another factor that influences the absorption of drugs in children is the irregularity in intestinal motility. The time to reach maximum blood concentration is longer, but the absorbed drug amount does not differ between immature organism and mature one as seen in the case of acetaminophen and oxazepam. The Absorption model may change considerably in the first weeks of extrauterine life due to changes in blood flow maturity, especially if it is accompanied by hypoxia. It is important to emphasize that the absorption of a drug could be increased or decreased depending on the physicochemical properties of the compound.

On the other hand, the intestinal mucus of the newborn can absorb large molecules such as proteins and this increase in the permeability is sometimes available for other chemical compounds. The decrease in the absorption speed is observed with some substances dependent on active transport. As the absorption of most drugs is by passive diffusion, the intestinal absorption in infants is comparable to that of adults. However, the action of a drug in infants could be more dangerous if the administration route is characterized by slow absorption instead of a route of fast absorption. When the absorption of a drug is fast, its elimination has little effect on its maximum concentration. In contrast, when the rate of absorption is slow, the maximum concentration depends on the ratio of absorption and elimination rates. The slower the elimination rates of a drug, the greater its blood concentration and the magnitude of the effect produced by a correct dose. Consequently, a drug administered through a slow absorption route at a given dose calculated according to the body weight, results in a higher concentration in infants than in adults for the fact that the rate of absorption is slower in the former. Hence, the likelihood that repeated administration of a substance would lead to toxic levels is higher when a fast absorption administration route is used, since the drug concentration would remain longer.

DISTRIBUTION

Following the absorption of drugs, they are distributed in all parts of the body by the bloodstream. Adequate distribution of drugs to the site of action depends primarily on characteristics like their liposolubility, the degree of their ionization and binding to plasma protein or to other specific tissues.

In the plasma, drugs usually bind to albumin. This union depends principally on the chemical structure of the drug and the nature of the binding formed with the protein. In other words, the distribution of a drug can be affected by qualitative and quantitative changes in plasma proteins and competition for the site of union with endogenous and exogenous compounds. Even though term newborns have plasma albumin at a value lower than that of adults, at a year old, their total proteins and plasma protein binding reaches the value of that of an adult.

The above is supported by various pharmacokinetic studies. For instance, in the binding of salicylates to plasma protein in the newborn, the fraction of free circulating drugs is increased. Juarez et al., demonstrated that the area under the curve of salicylates depends on the type and severity of the sickness in children with autoimmune diseases [13]. In the case of diazepam, the distribution is lower in newborns because of its high liposolubility and reduced body fat content of the newborns. The binding of phenobarbital to proteins is low and hence its volume of distribution is higher consequently, the concentration of the free drug is very high (60-64%) which reaches even a higher level in children with hyper-bilirubinemia. The differences in protein binding between newborns and adults may be due not only to the lower plasma protein concentrations, but also due to the differences in the qualitative properties of the binding [14]. For instance, some endogenous substances (fatty acids and hormones) may occupy binding sites in the first days of life and this leads to a reduction in the binding capacity.

The body composition varies with fetal development. The total body liquid decreases by approximately 76% of what it is at birth, which reflects a reduction in the amount of extracellular liquids [15]. Thus, water-soluble drugs have a greater distribution volume in early stages of development. In contrast, the distribution of liposoluble drugs as diazepam and thiopental vary depending on the fat content since in the fetus, the fat content is minimal.

Epidemiological studies have shown that adverse reactions to prednisone, phenytoin, and diazepam are more frequent in patients with hypoalbuminemia. Renal necrosis also leads to a reduction in the binding of drugs to proteins. Drug´s distribution volume (DV) is a hypothetic concept describing the space in which a drug is distributed. In the term newborn, the body liquid is divided into two compartments – intracellular and extracellular, and it is approximately 70% of the body weight, which decreases as the age of the child increases. The water-soluble drugs are generally distributed in both compartments and their concentrations in them depend only on their lipid/water partition coefficient and their binding rate to plasma proteins.

On the other hand, adipose tissue increases in the first two years of life, a fact that is important to consider when administering liposoluble drugs as Phenobarbital, which may be deposited in the fatty tissue and provoke toxicity. The increase in the distribution volume of water-soluble drugs results in a reduction in the maximum concentration and in the maximum effect. In virtue of such change in DV, the elimination half-life is prolonged. Consequently, in prolonged administration of a drug, the interval between doses should be longer in order to avoid excessive accumulation.

METABOLISM

The metabolism of most drugs usually takes place in the liver. In newborns, the cytochrome p-450-dependent oxidase enzymes of mixed function and conjugation enzymes are lower (50-70% less than that of adults). The formation of glucuronide per kilogram of body weight (essential for the functions of glucuronization) gets to adult values until the third or fourth year of age. For this, infants have a poor capacity to metabolize drugs, many of which have slow clearance and prolonged half-lives in the body. Table 3 shows some drugs whose half-life is altered in the infant. Therefore, the process of maturation should be considered when drugs are administered in this age group, especially if the drug is administered in prolonged form.

Table 3. Approximate average life of different drugs in newborns and adults

Drugs	Newborn age	Newborns (t1/2h)	Adults (t1/2h)
Acetaminophen		2.2 - 5	0.9 - 2.2
Diazepam		25 - 1000	40 - 50
Digoxin		60 - 70	30 - 60
Phenytoin	0 - 2 days	80	12 - 18
	3 - 14 days	18	
	14 - 50 days	6	
Phenobarbital	0 - 5 days	200	64 - 140
	5 - 15 days	100	
	1 - 30 months	50	
Salicylates		4.5 - 15	10 - 15
Theophylline	Newborn	13 - 26	5 - 10
	Children	3 - 4	

The newborns, particularly the premature, show a certain level of immaturity of the enzymatic systems responsible for normal metabolism and for biotransformation of drugs. For instance, several microsomal enzymes in the type 1 phase of metabolism, such as cytochrome p-450, hydroxylase and some esterases; and those that intervene in the conjugation of glucuronic acid in phase II metabolism do not exist or are in very small quantity. Thus, certain natural metabolites and some drugs have a very slow or null biotransformation in the newborns. Dealkylation reactions may be less altered for mepivacaine and diazepam as opposed to theophylline and caffeine, but n-methylation is the most affected step. In the postnatal stage, the enzymatic systems develop more rapidly. The majority of them reach the level of activity that is equal to that of adults between the first and the eighth week postpartum. Probably, all reaches their maximum activity in the first year of life.

Preschoolers, Schoolchidren and Adolescents

Although there are few studies carried out in these stages of life, most indicate that for several drugs, the children at these ages have an increased metabolic capacity [16]. For example, the metabolism of drugs was evaluated to determine the elimination half-life of theophylline, which undergoes demethylation through mixed oxidation functions. In the adolescents, a shorter elimination half-life than in adults was obtained. Similarly, it was found that children between one and eight years metabolize both antipyrine and phenylbutazone much more rapidly than adults. The same happens with acetaminophen.

Elimination

Most of the drugs administered are eliminated from the body either metabolized or unaltered by renal excretion. The renal excretion of drugs is less in the first stages of postnatal life because, on one part, the rate of drug arrival to the kidney is less. In the neonate, whose available water volume for drug distribution is higher, the concentration in the blood that irrigates the kidneys is lower. The blood volume, which passes through the kidney of an infant per unit of time is less in proportion to the total body water content. Because of the greater distribution volume and lower degree of blood supply, the filtration rate of drugs in the glomerulus of an infant is relatively slow, hence the mean elimination time of insulin in an infant is three times bigger than in an adult.

Immaturity in the elimination mechanisms of drugs in the infant has therapeutic repercussions. When the dosage is decided based on body size, the pharmacological action tends to prolong or increase or both. If the administration route is characterized by a faster rate of absorption, the concentration obtained at the site of action and the intensity of response will be normal. But if the drug levels last for a prolonged time, there is a risk of accumulation until toxic level if the time interval between one dose and another is not considered.

The importance of the maturity of glomerular filtration for the elimination of drugs is exemplified by the group of aminoglycoside antibiotics (kanamycin, gentamycin streptomycin) that are excreted unchanged. Their elimination half-lives in premature are more prolonged than in term newborns and both are more prolonged than in older children. The elimination of digoxin also depends on its glomerular excretion which is slowly cleared in newborn. The drugs like penicillin G and a good number of semisynthetic penicillin that depend on tissue secretion are slowly eliminated by the newborn. Their rates of excretion are directly related to postnatal age and reach adult values at three or four weeks of age. The comparison of premature babies with gestational ages of 30 to 33 weeks and infants small for gestational age showed a very similar excretion curve for ampicillin and both presented differences when compared with premature babies of the older gestational age of a range 34 to 35 weeks [17]. The regulation of acid-base equilibrium is not very efficient like in more advanced ages which may affect renal excretion of drugs. In older people, urine pH rhythmically changes during the 24 hours of the day in accordance with the period of sleep and awake. During the period of sleep, acid urine pH predominates and definitely, this would modify tubular reabsorption of drugs depending on their state of ionization. In less than one year old children, this rhythmic model of urine excretion is absent.

Failure to recognize that the elimination rate of a drug is altered in newborn may lead to subtherapeutic or excessive levels of the drug resulting in therapeutic failure or toxic effects. The elimination rate of drugs at a younger age could provoke accumulated toxic effects as seen with chloramphenicol that causes gray baby syndrome [18]. Conversely, fast elimination of a drug, in a standard therapeutic regimen, may give rise to insufficient drug concentration as seen in children that receive theophylline [19].

Dosification

To administrate the right dose of a drug to a child, it is necessary to consider individual variations in terms of genetic factors, disease process and clinical history. Until 15 or 20 years ago, the dose of a drug for children is empirically established using the rules that considered the age, weight, height or body surface. In this form, the doses were calculated for newborns as a fraction of the doses for the adults [20]. These somatic variables are related with different physiological functions that change with growth, which entails body weight (lean muscle mass), body height or body surface (basal metabolic rate). Though none of these rules is ideal to determine the doses that should be administered in newborns, the body surface seems to be the most adequate, because this variable has a better relation with some important physiological factors in the kinetic of some drugs [21]. The differences in the calculated doses depend on the method used. For instance, the ratio of body surface/weight in a term newborn is twice the value of that of an adult. Hence, the dose of a drug calculated in a newborn based on this ratio is twice as high as when calculated according to body weight.

Practically, there are no researches that evaluate the interaction between active growth and development processes and the specific pharmacological principles as well as the influence of the disease state. It is evident that due to the complexities of an organism in growth and development, it is very difficult to establish a well-defined base for the rational dosage of drugs. The immaturity and the general process of growth and development increase the potential risk of intoxication or therapeutic failure and this demands a better understanding of the problem in such a way that the current approach in which it is important to identify adverse effects should be directed at determining the optimal dose that improves efficacy and reduces the risk of toxicity.

Conclusion

The particular characteristics of children, especially the newborns, based on their changing body and physiological evolution, make them be considered as a particular population and as a group with a high risk for drug administration. Today, studies in pediatric clinical pharmacology, though limited worldwide, have continuously increased for being considered an area of risk.

There are numerous useful drugs for the adult and for the older children, but in which no studies have been performed in the newborns. Therefore, it is necessary to take into account the multiple changes that continuously occur in this stage of life when administering drugs to the newborns. It is pertinent to note that many drugs are approved and launched into the market without performing the necessary studies in children and in many occasions, may endanger the life of newborns. Thus, a physician must analyze the physiological aspects of the patient and the pharmacological aspects of the drug to be prescribed in order to select the therapeutic regimen that would lead to a rational management of the medicines. Sometimes, it will be necessary to request clinical studies that would support the decision of the physician in terms of the therapeutic scheme that he or she considers more adequate for the treatment of his/her pediatric patient so as to derive a better therapeutic response without forgetting the necessary precautions to ensure continuous risk-free management. The physician should be conscious of the changes of doses of the drugs determined by alterations in their processes of disposal at different ages. Also, he/she should be aware that adverse events of the drugs can become apparent even many years after.

References

[1] Gibaldi M, Perrier D. *Farmacocinética.* [Pharmacokinetics.] Barcelona, España: Ed Reverté; 2004. p.5.

[2] Hardman JG, Limbird LE, Gilman AG. *Goodman & Gilman's the pharmacological basis of Therapeutics.* 10th ed. New York: McGraw-Hill; 2001.

[3] Wagner JG. *Pharmacokinetics for the Pharmaceutical Scientist,* Lancaster, PA: Technomic Publishing Company, Inc; 1993.

[4] Nahata MC. Evolution of pediatric clinical pharmacy. *Ann Pharmacother.* 2006;40:1170-9.

[5] Gonçalves AC, Reis AM, Gusmão AC, Bouzada MC. Drug utilization profile in the neonatal unit of a university hospital: a prospective observational study in Brazil. *Int J Clin Pharm.* 2015;37:645-55.

[6] Krasowski MD, Penrod LE. Clinical decision support of therapeutic drug monitoring of phenytoin: measured versus adjusted phenytoin plasma concentrations. *BMC Med Inform Decis Mak.* 2012; 14;12:7.

[7] Carlos MA, Babyn PS, Marcon MA, Moore AM. Changes in gastric emptying in early postnatal life. *J Pediatr* 1997; 130:931-937.

[8] Pullen J, Driessen M, Stolk LM, Degraeuwe PL, van Tiel FH, Neef C, Zimmermann LJ. Amoxicillin pharmacokinetics in (preterm) infants aged 10 to 52 days: effect of postnatal age. *Ther. Drug Monit.* 2007;29:376-80.

[9] Yu G, Zheng QS, Li GF. Similarities and differences in gastrointestinal physiology between neonates and adults: a physiologically based pharmacokinetic modeling perspective. *AAPS J.* 2014;16:1162-6.

[10] Batchelor HK, Fotaki N, Klein S. Paediatric oral biopharmaceutics: key considerations and current challenges. *Adv. Drug Deliv. Rev.* 2014;73:102-26.

[11] Rodieux F, Gotta V, Pfister M, van den Anker JN. Causes and consequences of variability in drug transporter activity in pediatric drug therapy. *J Clin Pharmacol.* 2016;56 Suppl 7:S173-92.

[12] Schoen K, Yu T, Stockmann C, Spigarelli MG, Sherwin CM. Use of methylxanthine therapies for the treatment and prevention of apnea of prematurity. *Paediatr. Drugs.* 2014;16:169-77.

[13] Juárez Olguín H, Flores Pérez J, Lares Asseff I, Loredo Abdala A, Carvajal Rodríguez L. Comparative pharmacokinetics of ASA and its metabolites in children suffering from autoimmune disease. *Biopharma. Drug Dispos.* 2004;25:1-7.

[14] McNamara P, Alcorn J. Protein binding predictions in infants. *AAPS Pharm Sci* 2002; 4:1-8.

[15] Krasowski MD, Penrod LE. Clinical decision support of therapeutic drug monitoring of phenytoin: measured versus adjusted phenytoin plasma concentrations. *BMC Med Inform Decis Mak.* 2012; 14;12:7.

[16] Hattis D, Ginsberg G, Sonawane B. Differences in pharmacokinetics between children and adults—II. Children's variability in drug elimination half-lifes and in some parameters needed for physiologically-based pharmacokinetic modeling. *Risk Anal.* 2003; 23:117–42.

[17] Prober GCh, Stevenson KD, Benitz EW. The use of antibiotics neonates weighing less than 1200 grams. *Pediatr lnfect Dis J.* 1990; 9:111-21.

[18] Lares Al, Lugo GG, Pérez GG, Pérez OB, Guillé PA, Juárez OH. Predicción bayesiana de las concentraciones séricas de cloranfenicol en niños con sepsis y desnutrición. [Bayesian prediction of chloramphenicol plasma concentrations in children with sepsis and malnutrition] *Rev lnvest Clin* 1999; 51:159-65.

[19] Lowry JA, Jarrett RV, Wasserman G, Pettett G, Kauffman RE. Theophylline toxicokinetics in premature newborns. *Arch. Pediatr Adolesc. Med.* 2001;155:934-9.

[20] Dipiro JT, Spruill WJ, Wade WE, Blouin RA. Concepts in clinical pharmacokinetics. *Am Soc. Health-System Pharm.* 4 ed. 2005.

[21] McGinnity DF, Collington J, Austin RP, Riley RJ. Evaluation of human pharmacokinetics, therapeutic dose and exposure predictions using marketed oral drugs. *Curr. Drug Metab.* 2007; 8:463-79.

In: The Optimization of Drug Prescribing ... ISBN: 978-1-53612-263-3
Editor: Hugo Juarez Olguin

Chapter 5

PHARMACOLOGY FOR THE FETUS AND THE NEWBORN

***Hugo Juarez Olguín*[1,2,*] *and Ismael Lares-Asseff*[3]**

[1]Laboratorio de Farmacología, Instituto Nacional de Pediatría, México City, México

[2]Departamento de Farmacología, Facultad de Medicina, Universidad Nacional Autónoma de México. México

[3]Centro de Investigación Interdisciplinario para el Desarrollo Integral Regional, Instituto Politécnico Nacional, Durango, México

ABSTRACT

During intrauterine life, the fetus can be exposed to a series of substances ingested by the mother, some of which are necessary for her health but detrimental to the fetus. The noxious effects of such exposure could present in the fetus immediately after exposure or be manifested at the time of delivery and sometimes weeks after birth. The passage of drugs or nutrients across the placenta depends on physicochemical properties of the substances that enable them to cross the placenta barrier, and thus get in contact with the fetus and produce harmful effects.

* Corresponding Author Email: juarezol@yahoo.com

Considering the physicochemical properties of the substances, the possibility of such compounds to cross the placenta barrier and thence to the fetus can be predicted. Equally, it is important to consider the characteristics of the newborn as an immature being, different from adults, when carrying out pharmacokinetic and pharmacodynamic processes. Based on the latter, it is important to know the behavior or characteristics of the fetus and the newborn in the face of drug management and above all, consider the advantages and disadvantages of the use of such drugs for the care of a being yet in development, as described in this work.

Pharmacology During the Gestational Period

During intrauterine life, the fetus may be exposed to a series of drugs and toxic substances whose effects can be immediate and cause fetal death or produce some damage that may manifest at the moment of birth or even weeks, months or years later [1,2]. Establishing a relationship between intrauterine exposure to drugs and pathologic damage produced in the fetus has been difficult, unless such damage is confirmed after some time [3, 4].

The placenta forms a maternal-fetal interface starting from the moment the blastocyte is implanted in the uterus until the delivery of the product [5]. The primitive trophoblast acts as an anchoring device and satisfies the nutritional needs of the internal cell mass by phagocytosis of the maternal decidual tissue. In this developmental phase, the transport processes between the mother and the inner cell mass are started. When the trophoblast is differentiated and the cell mass is internalized in the embryo, the placenta – which originates in the embryo – adopts the roles of the organs not yet developed. Hence, its functions include the production of a wide range of substances that are essential to the growth and development of the fetus. The placenta is an organ with immense reserves that operates under a safety factor, which offers a safeguard environment to the fetus. This fact becomes clear by the birth of healthy children with a deficient placenta, which demonstrates that the placenta is able to maintain sufficiency of its functions and preserve the child unharmed [6, 7].

Several studies indicate that the number of layers which separate the maternal circulation from fetal circulation conditions the velocity with which substances are transported across the placenta. The thickness of the human placenta membranes ranges from 25 mm at the beginning of gestation to approximately 2 mm at its completion, which suggests that there are changes in the transference of compounds throughout pregnancy [8]. Some examples are shown in table 1.

Table 1. Pathological effects of drugs on the fetus and the newborn

Fetal emaciation
Teratogenesis
Carcinogenesis
Alteration of the reproductive system
Abnormal prenatal growth
Abnormal postnatal growth
Inadequacy for delivery process
Hematological disorders
Metabolic changes
Mental retardation
Neurological sequels

Factors Regulating Mother-Fetus Substance Exchange

Placental Transport Mechanisms

To be able to cross the placenta, substances follow certain basic transport mechanisms through biological membranes, especially simple diffusion mechanisms. Most drugs cross the placenta through this mechanism. The diffusion rate depends on a concentration gradient between maternal and fetal circulation, as well as on physicochemical properties of the substances, such as their lipid-solubility, degree of ionization and molecular weight [9, 10].

Compounds with a high degree of liposolubility are optimally transferred, due to the structural and physicochemical characteristics of membranes. In addition, transference is favored by non-ionized or low molecular weight compounds [11]. It is not adequate to extrapolate the mechanism through which some endogenous compounds such as glucose and possibly iron diffuse across the placenta to drug transport in this place. An important number of endogenous nutrients including amino acids, creatinine, sodium, calcium and phosphates cross the placenta against a concentration gradient, probably by means of active transport mechanisms however, very few drugs or other genobiotic agents have been shown to cross the placenta in this form [12].

Factors Regulating Placental Drug Transport

Lipid Solubility

As previously mentioned, highly lipid-soluble drugs rapidly cross the placenta with its passage only being limited by maternal blood flow within the placental lacunae. Drugs such as barbiturates, minor tranquilizers, narcotic analgesics and local anesthetics are transferred by this mechanism hence, they are known as flow-dependent [13]. The high permeability of the placenta to these drugs is reflected by their rapid transference. On administration of intravenous bolus of a drug with flow-dependent characteristics e.g., meperidine to a pregnant woman, the peak fetal umbilical venous concentration is reached very quickly [14].The reduction of the placental blood flow due to its decrease in uterine vessels produces a decrease in drug transference. This may occur, for example, as a result of normal uterine contractions during labor by the administration of oxytocic drugs [15]. Highly ionizable or non-lipid soluble drugs can be transferred in a limited way owing to low permeability of this biological barrier. The rate of crossing the placenta by these substances is not usually influenced by flow, as it occurs with lipid-soluble drugs.

Protein Binding

As previously mentioned, the transference of non-ionized and lipid-soluble drugs across the placenta is proportional to the maternal-fetal free drug concentration gradient. Therefore, the passage of drugs with high affinity to maternal plasma proteins will be delayed owing to the decrease in the available free drug concentration gradient. After crossing the placenta, the drugs bind to fetal plasma proteins, which act as transporters for some molecules that cross from the maternal circulation. The net effect of this phenomenon is a delay in equilibrating the drug concentration between the maternal and fetal circulations, since a relatively large amount has to be transferred, even with a low concentration gradient, for there to be a balance of the free drug in both circulations. In addition, there is a difference between maternal and fetal plasma drug binding [16]. For example, some drugs as antibiotics, local anesthetics, phenytoin and phenobarbital, show a high degree of maternal protein binding when compared with fetal protein binding which is exactly the opposite of what occurs with salicylates.

THE TRANSPORT OF SOME KEY SUBSTANCES

Glucose

Glucose is the most important metabolite required by the developing fetus. This is why some of the first investigations on placental transference in vivo were conducted to demonstrate the transference of this sugar. Its transport is known to occur by facilitated diffusion, mediated by specific carriers that favor the input of glucose towards the fetus [17].

Vitamins

Different transport systems across the microvilli membrane have been described for water-soluble vitamins as choline, ascorbic acid and riboflavin. Studies in human placenta show that choline transport occurs on both directions (maternal and fetal) of the synciotrophoblast [18].

Micronutrients and Iron

Fetal requirements of iron, about a total of 300 mg during pregnancy, are covered by transplacental iron transport from maternal transferrin. During pregnancy, in addition to including iron-rich foods in the diet, it is necessary to take iron supplement under the indication of a doctor. Most of the iron required during pregnancy is to increase the hemoglobin mass in the mother. This increase occurs in healthy pregnant women, who have sufficient iron reserves or are adequately supplemented with the mineral [19].

Insulin

It has been shown that insulin does not cross the placenta in significant amount in the humans. Recently, monoclonal antibodies have been used to confirm that placenta membranes contain different types of receptors for insulin and insulin-like growth factor (IGF) which function as important regulators of fetal growth, and IGF-1 and IGF-2 have been suggested to partially mediate this effect by promoting adequate development and functions of the placenta. For example, IGF-1 plasma levels are significantly decreased on day 21 in gestating rats on low-protein diets. Therefore, it can be speculated that decreased levels of maternal hormones, such as insulin, leptin and IGF-1, are signals associating maternal protein malnutrition with the main amino acid-transporters in the placenta. Compound-transference tendencies are driven by the biological requirements of each compartment. Table 2 shows the value levels of some compounds relating to each side of the compartment [20].

Table 2. Comparison of the levels of some compounds in their equilibrium state between the maternal and fetal compartments

	Equal	Lower in the fetus	Higher in the fetus
Amino acids		+	
Urea	+		
Uric acid	+		
Creatinine	+		
Inorganic			+
phosphorus		+	
Free fatty acids		+	
Cholesterol		+	
Glucose			+
Lactic acid			+
Calcium	+		
Magnesium	+		
Chlorine	+		
Sodium	+		
Potassium			+
Iron			
Vitamins	+		
Lipid soluble			+
Water soluble		+	
Chorionic			
gonadotropin		+	
Placental lactogen			+
Growth hormone			

DRUG PLACENTAL METABOLISM

Although the placenta is able to metabolize drugs, its contribution to transform xenobiotic agents is not yet well defined. Due to its reaction capacity, the human placenta, when compared with the liver, is an organ very much less active in the function of biotransformation in the last trimester of gestation. However, its contribution to the synthesis and degradation of endogenous substances, as steroid hormones, is very important especially the ones involving the participation of 1A1 and 2E1 enzymes [21, 22].

PHARMACOLOGY OF THE NEWBORN

Once a child is born, he or she is highly vulnerable to different unfavorable events. For instance, delivery, per se, is an act fraught with the possibility of complications, while the contact with his or her new environment and with micro-organisms are capable of producing changes and infections that may affect his or her development and growth. So at times, it becomes necessary to have recourse to drug administration. Due to the immaturity of the organs of the newborn, such drug administration is liable to pharmacokinetic effects different from that of adults and older children. For example, pharmacological processes such as absorption, distribution, metabolism and excretion by the newborn are usually lower [23,24], and so, this should be considered at the moment of making a prescription.

Drug Distribution

The composition of the body of a newborn evolves rapidly. Table 3 shows the relative weight evolution of different organs and tissues according to age. Neonates have a markedly more elevated percentage of water than humans of other ages (70% of body weight [25] in neonates and 80% in small premature neonates). With regard to extracellular water, 40% of the body weight of a newborn corresponds to this fluid and since many drugs are diffused through extracellular spaces with water as a vehicle to reach the receptor sites, changes in the body composition of an infant all along his or her development would invariably produce a change in drug distribution volumes. This is very important, especially in the case of water-soluble drugs, such as aminoglycosides.

In the case of body fat composition, approximately 0.5% of the total weight of a neonate is fat and this increases to a range of 15-20% at six months of age. Thereafter, the body fat composition gradually begins to decrease until adolescence. The body fat composition plays a vital role in the distribution of lipid-soluble drugs since these drugs tend to accumulate in the fatty tissues. Thus, organs that generally accumulate high concentrations of lipid-soluble drugs have to be considered when administering such drugs. Unlike adults with higher body fat composition, the organs of a newborn accumulate lower concentrations of lipid-soluble drugs, e.g., barbiturates and coumarinics. The end result of this is a delay in their serum clearance in the newborn and sequestration in the adults hence, the necessity of drug surveillance when these medicines are administered [26, 27].

Table 3. Percentage of total weight according to age*

Organ/tissue	Fetus	Full-term newborn	Adult
Skeletal muscle	25	25	40
Skin	13	4	6
Skeleton	22	18	14
Heart	0.6	0.5	0.4
Liver	4	5	2
Kidneys	13	12	2
Brain	12	12	2

* Organs and tissues relative weight according to age, expressed in percentage (%) of total body weight.

Absorption

Drug absorption in children is often similar to that in adults. However, this is always subject to the influence of certain factors as blood flow, gastrointestinal function, composition of gastrointestinal bacterial flora, vomiting, administration route and plasma protein binding.

Blood Flow

After an intramuscular or subcutaneous injection, absorption in neonates and adults is known to depend mainly on the blood flow rate to the injected muscles or subcutaneous area. In case of low muscular mass, if an injection is applied, absorption may be irregular and difficult to predict, since the drug will remain in the muscle and will be absorbed slower than expected. This aspect can be seriously compromised in neonates, owing to poor peripheral perfusion associated with lower cardiac output, as occurs in cases of cardiovascular shock, vasoconstriction by sympathomimetic drugs and heart failure, or due to some serious respiratory disease, as sometime seen in adults. If the risk decreases suddenly, there can be an immediate and unpredictable increase in the amount of drug entering the circulation, which can be a cause for the appearance of toxic concentrations. This situation is particularly common with drugs as cardiac glycosides [28], antibiotics [29, 30], aminoglycosides and anticonvulsants [31-33]. Increasing the distribution volume can alter pharmacokinetics and tissue penetration, as well as the clearance of drugs such as indomethacin and vancomycin. In the presence of these situations, drug monitoring and dose adjustments are recommended to avoid possible toxic effects or treatment failures.

Gastrointestinal Function

Gastrointestinal system in neonates exhibits important biochemical and physiological differences in comparison with older people. For instance, the production and secretion of gastric acids are directly related to the weight and gestational age in neonates. At birth, pH usually ranges from 6 - 8; while gastric acidity increases within the first 10 days after birth. In premature infants, gastric acid secretion is slower than in full-term infants and this implies the presence of larger amount of ionizable compounds that are more difficult to absorb.

During the neonatal period, gastric emptying time is prolonged from 6 to 8 h on the first day of life, and the frequency is directly affected by the presence of food, its amount and consistency. For example, liquid-consistent and sugary food will delay gastric emptying. Therefore, the absorption of drugs administered by oral route will be faster in neonates, with peak absorption time of a few minutes, when there is a delay in gastric emptying caused, for example, by some acidic food.

Composition of Gastrointestinal Bacterial Flora

This is another factor that modifies drug absorption, since it influences on intestinal motility, as well as on nutrients, bile salts and drug metabolism. Bacterial flora depends on patient's postnatal age, type of delivery, type of diet and on the pharmacotherapy used. Metabolic capability and bacterial microflora function are low in the newborn, since optimal degree of maturation has not been achieved, and which will not be reached until 4 years of age. Drugs that are absorbed in the small bowel can have its absorption and therapeutic effect delayed because peristalsis in the neonate is irregular and generally slows. Therefore, the amount of drug absorbed in the small bowel can be unpredictable. If peristalsis is slow, a higher amount of the drug is absorbed and this may provoke toxicity in the patient. Conversely, an increase in peristalsis, as in diarrheic conditions, may cause lower absorption due to a decrease in intestinal surface area.

Vomiting

Newborns are susceptible to constant vomiting or spitting up. Undoubtedly, this can influences on oral drugs absorption in the newborn.

Table 4 shows the differences in the oral absorption of some drugs in the neonate as compared with older children [25].

Table 4. Oral absorption (bioavailability) of different drugs in the neonate in comparison with older children and adults

Drug	Absorption in the neonate
Penicillin G	Higher
Ampicillin	Higher
Phenylbutazone	Higher
Phenytoin	Lower
Phenobarbital	Lower
Acetaminophen	Lower
Nalidixic acid	Lower
Rifampicin	Lower
Diazepam	Equal
Digoxin	Equal
Sulfonamides	equal

Administration Route

Due to their physiological characteristics, different routes of drug administration are used in newborns. For example, the most adequate route for chloramphenicol in this age group is intramuscular, since adequate therapeutic serum concentrations are not reached with the oral route. On the other hand, the topical route is frequently used in pediatrics. The skin is an entrance door for different micro-organisms that cause local and systemic infections. In neonates, particularly when premature, the skin can easily be damaged or injured owing to the large amount of water it contains. These patients are more exposed to suffer infections by bacteria and fungi, which increases the risk of triggering toxic effects due to topical application of substances. Total skin surface area ratio of the newborn with regard to weight is, in turn, approximately 3 times bigger than in adults.

Consequently, topical drug bioavailability is approximately 3-fold higher in newborns than in adults. There are very clear examples of different toxic substances the newborn is exposed to. Among these, laundry detergents with pentachlorophenol and hydrocortisone in the cases of diaper dermatitis can be mentioned.

Another route through which a newborn can receive some drugs is the breast milk. If during breast feeding a mother is ingesting a medication that is excreted through breast milk, obviously, the medication will be passed over to the child [34, 35]. The newborn may be exposed to adverse effects of drugs that are excreted through breast milk (> 10%) and therefore, monitoring of the neonate is important when he is being breastfed. For example, doxefin (miconazole/tinidazole) is excreted into breast milk, and even if the mother takes small doses of the drug, it crosses to her child and this may provoke numerous adverse effects as vomiting, navicular abdomen and muscular hypotonia in the newborn and at times, this may require hospitalization [36, 37].

Plasma Protein Binding

Albumin is the protein with more drug fixation and transport properties. In neonates, binding to proteins is much lower than in older people. Some studies on plasma albumin and α-1a acid glycoprotein variability in healthy neonates and neonates with renal failure and liver dysfunction show that, as liver dysfunction progresses, albumin concentration decreases, thus resulting in higher amounts of free drug being present, whereas glycoprotein concentration remains unchanged. However, there is no correlation between the levels of albumin and glycoproteins and bilirubin concentrations in patients with liver disease, which, in addition to being an indicator of hepatic function for drug metabolism, it is also an indicator to know any possible interaction at the level of protein binding due to displacement between two or more compounds with high affinity to proteins. The clinician should consider this affinity to proteins before prescribing any drug and avoid, as much as possible, concurrent use of such compounds at early ages.

Table 5 shows the binding degree of some drugs to plasma proteins, which depends on age-related variables, such as absolute amount of available proteins and their binding sites, drug-protein affinity constancy, the pathophysiological condition and the presence of competing endogenous substances for the proteins [25]. Protein binding is reflected on distribution volume and body clearance of the drug. Some drugs compete with albumin-bound bilirubin. If serum bilirubin increases due to physiological reasons or blood type incompatibility, it can displace the drug from albumin and increase its free concentration, and thus produces toxicity. An example of this phenomenon is what happens with phenytoin administration, an anticonvulsant drug [38, 39].

Acid-natured drugs such as salicylates and sulphonamides are slowly eliminated from the neonate, since they displace bilirubin from its point of fixation to serum albumin [40, 41]. This produces an increase of free albumin, a situation that enables its passage across the blood-brain barrier in a higher concentration and this can produce cerebral lesion. Interactions by displacement of plasma protein binding sites produce dramatic conditions in the newborn. For example, if plasma protein binding of a drug decreases from 99 to 98%, the result is a two-fold increase (from 1 to 2%) in the drug concentration which can result in a toxic effect.

Table 5. Plasma protein binding of selected drugs in newborns and adults

Drug	Plasma protein binding	
	Neonates*	Adults*
Paracetamol	36.8	47.5
Chloramphenicol	31.0	42.0
Morphine	46.0	66.0
Phenobarbital	32.4	50.7
Phenytoin	74.4	85.8
Promethazine	69.8	82.7

* Average binding values (%).

METABOLISM

Drug metabolism occurs mainly in the liver. In the neonate, the concentration of mixed function cytochrome P450 dependent oxidase enzymes and conjugation enzymes is 50-70% of the level in adults. Glucuronic acid formation does not reach adult values until the third or fourth year of life. Therefore, neonates have little capability to metabolize drugs, many of which have slow clearance and prolonged half-life. Pharmacokinetics studies of lidocaine show that infants younger than 1 month and low birth weight exhibit elevated distribution values and longer half-life, indicating that treatment regimens should be reduced in this group of patients [42].

ELIMINATION

Drug excretion or elimination is a very important factor. Glomerular filtration rate (GFR) is much lower in infants born before 34 weeks of gestation than in full-term newborns, and lower in the later when with respect to older infants, children or adults (Table 6). The rate is calculated based on the body surface area and in full-term newborns, its value is only 30 or 40% of adult value. The function improves in the first week of life, during which GFR and renal plasma flow are increased by 50%; by the third week it increases to 50-60% of the adult value; and from 6 to 12 months, they level up to adult values. Therefore, drugs depending on renal function for elimination are slowly cleared from the body during the first weeks of life.

The group of drugs whose clearance is altered includes penicillins, which are cleared in premature newborns at 34% with respect to the rate in adults for body weight. Consequently, the dose of this group of drugs should be reduced at that proportion in this group of infants. A decrease in renal elimination rate has also been observed for aminoglycosides (amikacin, gentamicin, neomycin and streptomycin) in neonates due to immaturity of the organ responsible for this function. Pharmacokinetics studies of the antiviral zidovudine in newborns with AIDS show that elimination is slow at birth and gradually increases within the first week of life, reaching a plateau between the fourth and the eight weeks of age. Zidovidine bioavailability increases in children younger than 14 days of age due to a decrease of first step metabolism, i.e., the metabolism a drug undergoes before reaching the systemic circulation, understood as the body's capability to clear the drug from blood; hence the agreement of some authors to call it clearance.

Table 6. Growth factors affecting renal excretion of drugs

Physiological variables	Effect on		
	Newborns	Infancy	Childhood
Renal flow	Increased or decreased	Increased	Present
Urinary circadian rhythm	Absent	Present	Normal
Glomerular filtration	Decreased	Decreased or normal	Normal
Tubular secretion	Decreased	Normal	Normal
Tubular reabsorption	Decreased	Increased, decreased or normal	Normal
Urinary pH	Acid	Variable	Variable

CONCLUSION

Owing to the changing body and physiological evolution of newborns, they should be considered a particular and high-risk population when administering drugs. There are countless drugs that are useful for adults or older children however, these drugs have not been subjected to pharmacological studies for their rational administration to newborns, which is extremely necessary, especially when we take into account that this population continuously suffer multiple changes. It should be pointed out that many drugs are approved and launched into the market without performing the necessary trials in children, and many times they can put the life of the newborn in danger.

REFERENCES

[1] Šlamberová, R. Drugs in pregnancy: the effects on mother and her progeny. *Physiol. Res.* 2012; 61 Suppl 1:S123-35.

[2] Aiken, C. E., Aiken, A. R., Cole, J. C., Brockelsby, J. C., Bamber, J. H. Maternal and fetal outcomes following unplanned conversion to general anesthetic at elective cesarean section. *J. Perinatol.* 2015; 35: 695-9.

[3] Hodge, L. S., Tracy, T. S. Alterations in drug disposition during pregnancy: implications for drug therapy. *Expert Opin. Drug Metab. Toxicol.* 2007; 3:557-71.

[4] Gokhale, S. G., Panchakshari, M. B. Maternal medication causing drug dystonia in a newborn: placental transfer of drugs. *J. Matern. Fetal. Neonatal. Med.* 2004; 16:215-7.

[5] Shiverick, K. T., Slikker, W. Jr., Rogerson, S. J., Miller, R. K. Drugs and the placenta: a workshop report. *Placenta.* 2003; 24 Suppl A: S55-9.

[6] Jauniaux, E., Gulbis, B. In vivo investigation of placental transfer early in human pregnancy. *Eur. J. Obstet. Gynecol. Reprod. Biol.* 2000; 92:45-9.

[7] Punshon, T., Chen, S., Finney, L., Howard, L., Jackson, B. P., Karagas, M. R., Ornvold, K. High-resolution elemental mapping of human placental chorionic villi using synchrotron X-ray fluorescence spectroscopy. *Anal. Bioanal. Chem.* 2015; 407:6839-50.

[8] van der Aa, E. M., Peereboom-Stegeman, J. H., Noordhoek, J., Gribnau, F. W., Russel, F. G. Mechanisms of drug transfer across the human placenta. *Pharm. World Sci.* 1998; 20:139-48.

[9] Stepensky, D. Prediction of drug disposition on the basis of its chemical structure. *Clin. Pharmacokinet.* 2013; 52:415-31.

[10] Włoch, S., Pałasz, A., Kamin´ ski, M. Active and passive transport of drugs in the human placenta. *Ginekol. Pol.* 2009; 80:772-7.

[11] Vähäkangas, K., Myllynen, P. Drug transporters in the human blood placental barrier. *Br. J. Pharmacol.* 2009; 158:665-78.

[12] Gedeon, C., Koren, G. Designing pregnancy centered medications: drugs which do not cross the human placenta. *Placenta.* 2006; 27:861-8.

[13] Eshkoli, T., Sheiner, E., Ben-Zvi, Z., Holcberg, G. Drug transport across the placenta. *Curr. Pharm. Biotechnol.* 2011; 12:707-4.

[14] Giaginis, C., Theocharis, S., Tsantili-Kakoulidou, A. Current toxicological aspects on drug and chemical transport and metabolism across the human placental barrier. *Expert Opin. Drug Metab. Toxicol.* 2012; 8:1263-75.

[15] Ganapathy, V., Prasad, P. D., Ganapathy, M. E., Leibach, F. H. Placental transporters relevant to drug distribution across the maternal-fetal interface. *J. Pharmacol. Exp. Ther.* 2000; 294:413-20.

[16] Nanovskaya, T. N., Patrikeeva, S., Hemauer, S., et al. Effect of albumin on transplacental transfer and distribution of rosiglitazone and glyburide. *J. Matern. Fetal. Neonatal. Med.* 2008; 21:197-207.

[17] Pollex, E. K., Hutson, J. R. Genetic polymorphisms in placental transporters: implications for fetal drug exposure to oral antidiabetic agents. *Expert. Opin. Drug Metab. Toxicol.* 2011; 7:325-39.

[18] American Academy of Pediatrics Committee on Fetus and Newborn. Controversies concerning vitamin K and the newborn. American Academy of Pediatrics Committee on Fetus and Newborn. *Pediatrics.* 2003; 112:191-2.

[19] Klaassen, C. D., Aleksunes, L. M. Xenobiotic, bile acid, and cholesterol transporters: function and regulation. *Pharmacol. Rev.* 2010; 62:1-96.

[20] Juárez-Olguín, H., Lares-Asseff, I. Antecedentes farmacológicos gestacionales implicados con la etapa neonatal. Factores que regulan el intercambio de sustancias madre-feto. *Acta Pediátrica de México.*

1999; 20:250-6. [Gestational pharmacological antecedents involved with the neonatal stage. Factors that regulate the exchange of maternal-fetal substances. *Acta Pediátrica de México*. 1999; 20:250-6.]

[21] Zhu, Y., Song, X., Han, F., Li, Y., Wei, J., Liu, X. Alteration of histone acetylation pattern during long-term serum-free culture conditions of human fetal placental mesenchymal stem cells. *PLoS One*. 2015; 10(2):e0117068.

[22] Syme, M. R., Paxton, J. W., Keelan, J. A. Drug transfer and metabolism by the human placenta. *Clin. Pharmacokinet.* 2004; 43:487-514.

[23] Juárez Olguín, H., Sandoval Ramires, E., Guille Perez, A. Comportamiento del proceso LADME de los medicamentos en los niños. *Acta Pediátrica de México*. 2009; 30:23-30. [Behavior of the LADME process of medications in children. *Acta Pediátrica de México*. 2009; 30:23-30]

[24] Della-Giustina, K., Chow, G. Medications in pregnancy and lactation. *Emerg. Med. Clin. North. Am.* 2003; 21:585-613.

[25] Perez-Guille, G., Guille-Perez, A., Camacho-Vieyra, A., Juárez-Olguín, H., Lares Asef, I. Las directrices que rigen la terapéutica farmacológica en el recién nacido. *Perinatología y Reproducción Humana*. 2000; 14:22-31. [The guidelines of the pharmacological therapy in the newborn. *Perinatología y Reproducción Humana*. 2000; 14:22-31]

[26] Sørensen, H. T., Johnsen, S. P., Larsen, H., Pedersen, L., Nielsen, G. L., Møller, M. Birth outcomes in pregnant women treated with low-molecular-weight heparin. *Acta Obstet. Gynecol. Scand.* 2000; 79:655-9.

[27] Yurdakök, M. Fetal and neonatal effects of anticoagulants used in pregnancy: a review. *Turk. J. Pediatr.* 2012; 54:207-15.

[28] Qasqas, S. A., McPherson, C., Frishman, W. H., Elkayam, U. Cardiovascular pharmacotherapeutic considerations during pregnancy and lactation. *Cardiol. Rev.* 2004; 12:201-21.

[29] Einarson, A., Shuhaiber, S., Koren, G. Effects of antibacterials on the unborn child: what is known and how should this influence prescribing. *Paediatr. Drugs.* 2001; 3:803-16.

[30] Reali, A., Ximenes, A., Cuzzolin, L., Fanos, V. Antibiotic therapy in pregnancy and lactation. *J. Chemother.* 2005; 17:123-30.

[31] Cummings, C., Stewart, M., Stevenson, M., Morrow, J., Nelson, J. Neurodevelopment of children exposed in utero to lamotrigine, sodium valproate and carbamazepine. *Arch. Dis. Child.* 2011; 96:643-7.

[32] Holmes, L. B., Mittendorf, R., Shen, A., Smith, C. R., Hernandez-Diaz, S. Fetal effects of anticonvulsant polytherapies: different risks from different drug combinations. *Arch. Neurol.* 2011; 68:1275-81.

[33] Juárez Olguín, H., Lugo Goytia, G., Flores Murrieta, F., Ruiz García, M., Lares Asseff, I. Effect of treatment and additional disease on pharmacokinetics of valproic acid in children with epilepsy. *Rev. Inv. Clin.* 2010; 62:516-23.

[34] Chen, L., Liu, F., Yoshida, S., Kaneko, S. Is breast-feeding of infants advisable for epileptic mothers taking antiepileptic drugs? *Psychiatry Clin. Neurosci.* 2010; 64:460-8.

[35] Menon, S. J. Psychotropic medication during pregnancy and lactation. *Arch. Gynecol. Obstet.* 2008; 277:1-13.

[36] Reali, A., Ximenes, A., Cuzzolin, L., Fanos, V. Antibiotic therapy in pregnancy and lactation. *J. Chemother.* 2005; 17:123-30.

[37] Gentile, S. The safety of newer antidepressants in pregnancy and breast feeding. *Drug Saf.* 2005; 28:137-52.

[38] Joung, K. E., Cataltepe, S. U., Michael, Z., Christou, H., Mantzoros, C. S. Cord blood adipocyte fatty acid-binding protein levels correlate with gestational age and birth weight in neonates. *J. Clin. Endocrinol. Metab.* 2017; 102:1606-1613.

[39] Sethi, P. K., White, C. A., Cummings, B. S., Hines, R. N., Muralidhara, S., Bruckner, J. V. Ontogeny of plasma proteins, albumin and binding of diazepam, cyclosporine, and deltamethrin. *Pediatr. Res.* 2016; 79:409-15.

[40] Antonucci, R., Zaffanello, M., Puxeddu, E., Porcella, A., Cuzzolin, L., Pilloni, MD. Use of non-steroidal anti-inflammatory drugs in pregnancy: impact on the fetus and newborn. *Curr. Drug Metab.* 2012; 13:474-90.

[41] Burdan, F., Szumilo, J., Klepacz, R. Maternal toxicity of nonsteroidal anti-inflammatory drugs as an important factor affecting prenatal development. *Reprod. Toxicol.* 2009; 28:239-44.

[42] Cavalli Rde, C., Lanchote, V. L., Duarte, G., Dantas, E. C., de Prado, M. F., de Duarte LB. Pharmacokinetics and transplacental transfer of lidocaine and its metabolite for perineal analgesic assistance to pregnant women. *Eur. J. Clin. Pharmacol.* 2004; 60:569-74.

In: The Optimization of Drug Prescribing … ISBN: 978-1-53612-263-3
Editor: Hugo Juarez Olguin

Chapter 6

PHARMACOKINETIC PRINCIPLES IN THE USE OF ANTIBIOTICS IN PEDIATRICS

María-Gabriela Pérez Guille[1,*], Ismael Lares-Asseff[2] and Alejandra Toledo López[1]

[1]Department of Pharmacology. Instituto Nacional de Pediatria. Mexico City, Mexico

[2]Department of Pharmacogenetics, Instituto Politécnico Nacional. CIIDIR-Unidad Durango, Durango, México

ABSTRACT

One of the challenges in the field of pediatric infectology is how to make a potent antibiotic drug to arrive at the site of infection in active form and inadequate concentration throughout the time required for the drug to exercise its action. In addition, the antibiotic must not interfere with the host´s natural defense mechanism, such as phagocytosis and must be cleared from the body once it has completed its task, since its long-term permanence increases the risk of toxicity. In this chapter, the experience of three clinical cases is presented.

---

*Corresponding Author Email: reparo_gaby@yahoo.com.mx

BACKGROUND

The selection of an antibiotic is fraught with a series of questions which the clinician have to answer in order choose the appropriate dosage and dosage intervals that would yield therapeutic success. The main questions are: how should the antibiotic be administeredby continuous intravenous infusion or bolus injection at defined intervals? How often must it be administered and in what amount? Is it useful to know, in case of oral administration, if the patient should be given the drug on an empty stomach or with food? How many times a day should the drug be administered? What is the therapeutic range of a specific antibiotic for a specific infectious process? This knowledge is what would guide the establishment of optimum treatment regimen [1].

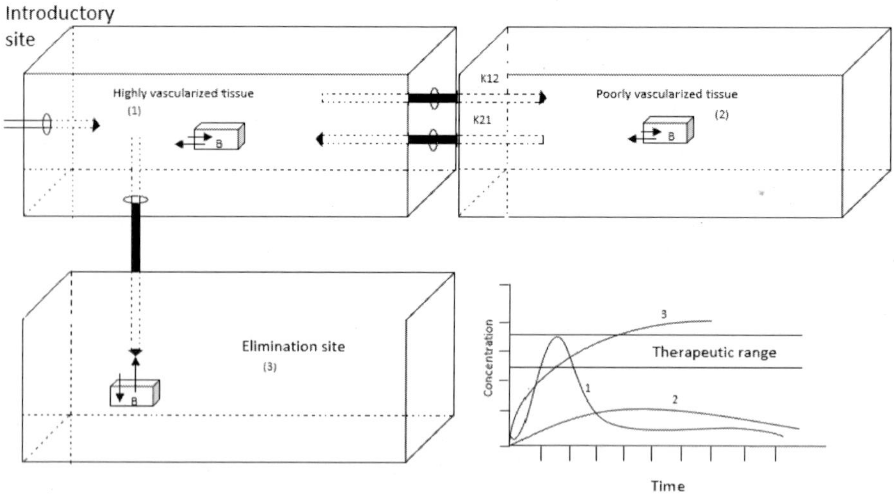

Figure 1. The compartmental model that exemplifies with bi-directional arrows the transfer rates of a drug between different compartments. The biophase (B) can be considered as the compartment that contains the receptors and can be found anywhere in the body. The curves of the graph show the temporal evolution of the concentrations in the different compartments - the central compartment (1), peripheral compartment (2) and organs of elimination (3).

Table 1. The formulas of the left column are applicable when the experimental data correspond to a mono-exponential model, while the formulas of the right side are used when the experimental data conform to a bio-exponential model

Pharmacokinetic Parameters	
One-compartment open Model	Two-compartment open Model
$t1/2_{el} = \frac{0.693}{kel}$	$t1/2_{\beta} = \frac{0.693}{\beta}$
$\frac{Vd}{C°p} = D$	$\frac{Vd\beta}{A + B} = D$
$CL_T = Kd.Vd$	$CL_T = \beta.Kd.Vd_{\beta}$
$\overline{C}_{EE} = \frac{K0(1-e^{-ke.t})}{CL_T}$	$\overline{C}_{EE} = \frac{K0(1-e^{-\beta.t})}{CL_T}$

Therefore, the aim of antibiotic therapy lies on achieving adequate concentrations, for a sufficient time, at the site of physiological action, defined as biophase, which is the body compartment containing the receptors for the antibiotic [2]. In the case of infectious diseases, the bacteria are the receptors of the antibiotics. As the infections occur in different parts of the body, the properties of the biophase may vary with the type of infection [3]. Thus, the biophase may have the characteristics of a deeper compartment, in which there is a slow balance of the drug, or be located in the superficial compartment, where the balance in the concentrations of the antibiotic is faster (Figure 1).

To answer the questions previously formulated, the optimization of the dosage regimens for the treatment of infectious diseases with antibacterial agents is extremely necessary, and for this, the physician is required to know the pharmacokinetic and pharmacodynamic parameters of the drug to be used, at least those which are important and optimal for the establishment of multiple treatment regimens. These parameters are the elimination half-life ($t^1/_2el$), the volume of distribution (VD), the total body clearance (CL_T) and the steady-state average concentration (C_{EE}). Ideally, these parameters are obtained from a pharmacokinetic study of the patient after having received a single dose of the drug or from a study performed in subjects with similar biological or pathological characteristics (Table 1). When the pharmacokinetic parameters are not possible to obtain directly from the patient, recourse is made to reports on studies in other subjects with similar biological and/or pathological characteristics that are published in the respective literature.

The pharmacokinetic parameters required for the evaluation and design of a treatment regimen (Table 1) is obtained from the decay curve of drug plasma concentrations as a function of time (Figure 2).

As observed in the curves of Figure 2, once the experimental data are adjusted to the best kinetic model that explains their behavior in the organism, according to the number of exponential phases, the values of the slope of terminal phase, represented by the elimination rate constant (Kel), are obtained when it is mono-exponential decay phase corresponding to one-compartment open model (graph a, Figure 2). Also, the values of the slope of terminal phase can be obtained from the constant (β) if the rate of loss of the drug in the organism is bi-exponential, which corresponds to two-compartment open model (graph b, Figure 2).

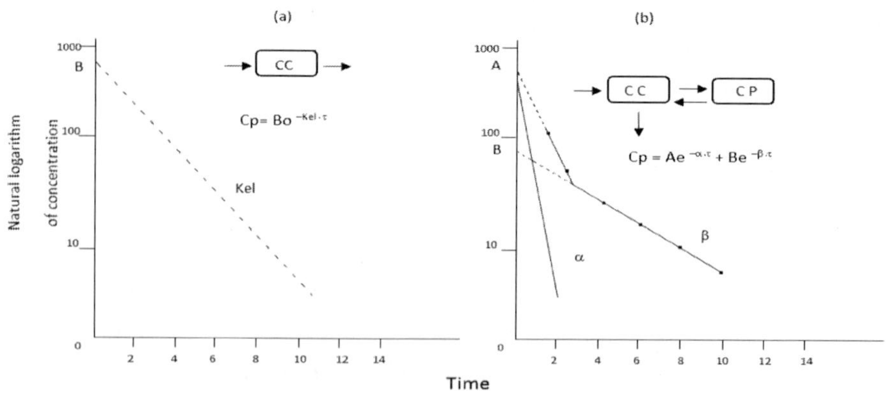

Figure 2. Semi-logarithmic curves of plasma concentration decay of a drug as a function of time whose behavior corresponds to an open compartment model (a) and to a bi-compartment model (b). In the upper right corner of both curves, the compartmental model is presented, with the general equation describing the kinetic behavior for each model, according to the number of exponential phases.

As seen in Figure 3, when the number of exponential phases defined in the slope of the plasma concentration over time, has more than two exponentials, then the model that would explain such behavior will be defined by a multi-compartment system. Therefore, the mathematical expressions of pharmacokinetics will be based on the kinetic model that conceives the organism as a compartmental system. Thus, the plasma concentrations of an intravenously administered drug for a mono-compartmental model can be described with an exponential equation:

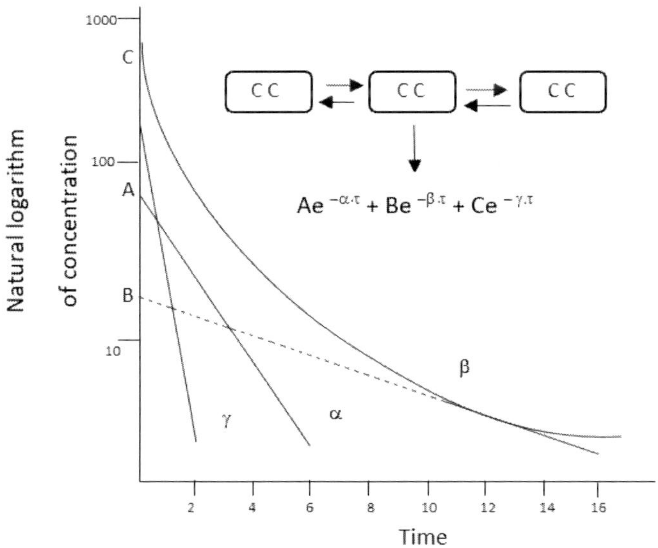

Figure 3. Semi-logarithmic curve that shows the temporal course of the plasma concentrations of a drug whose behavior is defined by an open three-compartment model (OTCM). In the upper right corner, the compartmental model is presented with the general equation describing the kinetic behavior.

$$Cp = B.e^{-Kel\,t} \qquad \text{(Eq. 1)}$$

Where Cp represents the concentration of the drug at any time. The value B is the intercept of the extrapolable slope to the ordinate and corresponds to the concentration at time zero. The value of e is the base of the natural logarithms raised to power –Kel.t, with t being the time elapsed and Kel the elimination rate constant which is characteristic for each drug.

The plasma concentrations as a function of time for a bi-compartmental model can be described with the exponential equation:

$$Cp= Ae^{-\alpha.t} + Be^{-\beta.t} \quad \text{(Eq. 2)}$$

Where A is the intercept of the distribution phase and B the intercept of elimination phase extrapolated to the ordinate, α and β are the distribution and elimination rate constants respectively and the value of e corresponds to the base of the natural logarithm raised to power $-\alpha.t$ for the second exponential phase.

Application of Pharmacokinetic in Clinical Practice

Pharmacokinetic of Multiple Doses

The administration of a treatment regimen in clinical practice requires the intermittent delivery of a constant dose at different intervals over a given period and must be sufficient to maintain the effective concentrations within the therapeutic index or within the therapeutic window during the time required to control the infectious process. The therapeutic window depends on the susceptibility of the microorganism involved in the infectious process to a specific antibiotic as well as on the maximum tolerance shown by the patient.

After the first administration (Figure 4), each new dose represents a greater increase in the previously achieved plasma concentrations, since the new concentration starts from the concentration amount of the previously administered drug remaining in the organism that has not yet been eliminated at the time of the administration of the new dose.

After multiple administrations, once the eliminated amount in the organism in the interval between doses is equal to the amount introduced in each administration, an equilibrium or peak concentration known as steady state is reached. In this state, in spite of the drug being administered, its concentrations in the blood are maintained within certain limits related to the dose and the interval between doses. The average concentrations in the steady state (C_{EE}) can be calculated by the following equation:

$$C_{EE}=\frac{Ko(1-e^{-kel.t})}{CL_T} \quad \text{(Eq.3)}$$

Where Ko is the fraction of the administered dose per unit of time and CL_T is the clearance of the drug that expresses the ability of the organism to eliminate it.

On obtaining the pharmacokinetic parameters corresponding to the elimination rate constant (Kel) as well as that of clearance or total clearance (CL_T) after performing a kinetic study of an antibiotic, such values are substituted in equation 3 to predict the concentrations in a steady state. Once this concentration is determined, we are now in condition to evaluate the therapeutic success.

EVALUATION OF THE SUCCESS OF A TREATMENT REGIMEN

In order to evaluate the therapeutic success from the point of view of pharmacokinetic, the phenomenon of drug accumulation must be taken into account until the average concentration in the steady state (C_{EE}) is reached.

This steady state is generally reached after five half-lives [4]. Thus, depending on the elimination half-life, the steady state is reached at different times for each antibiotic. For instance, if the elimination half-life of gentamycin, measured in a child, corresponds to 3.0 hours, the steady state for this aminoglycoside in this particular patient will be reached after 15 hours (3.0 X 5 = 15).

If the predicted concentrations in the beginning of the treatment fall within the desired therapeutic window, the probability of success is huge and this could be corroborated by measuring the concentrations of the antibiotics in the steady state.

In case the predicted plasma concentrations do not reach or exceed the therapeutic window, the treatment regimen is inadequate, since in the first case, the physician runs the risk of therapeutic failure and in the second case, the likelihood of toxicity will increase as the predicted levels increasingly exceed the maximum concentration. According to the mentioned criteria, it is interesting from the therapeutic point of view to define two concepts that will help to evaluate and design a new therapeutic regimen. These concepts are accuracy and precision.

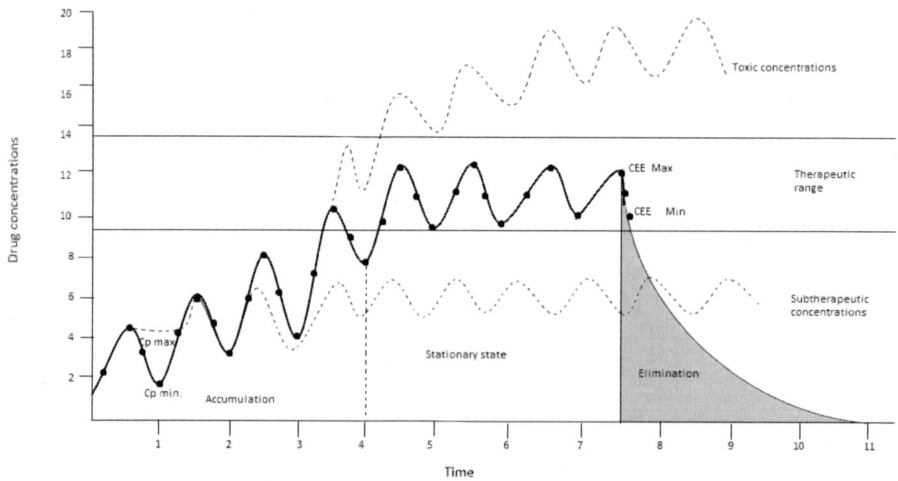

Figure 4. Representation of the accumulation of plasma concentration when a drug is repeatedly administered at regular intervals by oral route. Also, the elimination curve on suspending the treatment is observed. According to the treatment regimen, the concentrations in a steady state may correspond to toxic or subtherapeutic concentrations depending on whether if it is above or below the therapeutic window.

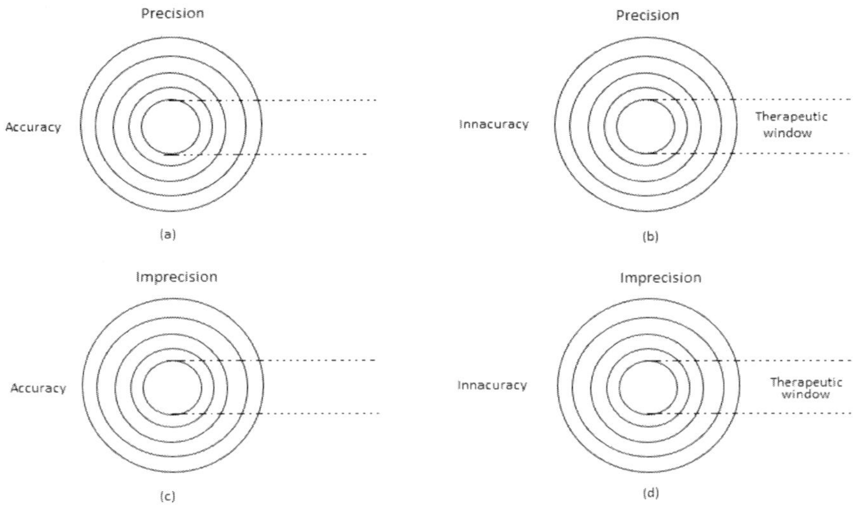

Figure 5. The target (central point of a field of fire) represents, in this case, the therapeutic window of a medicine. A dosage regimen should be designed just as if it were the target of a shooting point. Target a: If the concentrations are within the therapeutic index or the target and these are also grouped, as in this case, then there is accuracy and precision. Target b: If the concentrations are outside the therapeutic index but grouped, as in this case, then there is precision but inaccuracy. Target c: If the concentrations are within the therapeutic index but dispersed, as in this case, then there is imprecision and accuracy in the target. Target d: If the concentrations are outside the therapeutic index and dispersed all over the target, as in this case, then there is imprecision and inaccuracy.

From the practical point of view, these concepts and their interrelations are illustrated in Figure 5. Accordingly, the term "accuracy" should be used in medical therapeutics as a measure of the degree to which the concentrations obtained are in agreement with the concentrations within the therapeutic index, i.e., the desired therapeutic window.

The term "precision" describes the reproducibility of the concentrations within the desired therapeutic index. It is also considered as a measure of dispersion of concentration determined under the same condition within a dose regimen in the same subject and the same hour of the day.

The aim is to achieve the therapeutic objective of a treatment regimen corresponding to the desired pharmacological effect, which is obtained within a range of concentration called therapeutic window, which in turn is a function of both minimum inhibitory concentration of a microorganism to an antibiotic and assessed maximum tolerance. On establishing a treatment regimen, we are practically aiming to make our shot hit a target, which in this case is the therapeutic window. To achieve therapeutic success, it is required to be accurate and at the same time precise. Accuracy and precision should be maintained for a sufficient time to achieve the desired therapeutic effect. For this, the physician is required to know the rate of drug clearance and to control the rate of entry so that drug concentrations reach equilibrium within the desired therapeutic window.

Optimization of Treatment Regimen

When the therapeutic concentrations are required to be reached immediately, a loading dose (LD) is calculated from the following formula:

$$LD = \frac{1.44.\ MD.\ t1/2el}{T} \quad \text{(Eq.4)}$$

The maintenance dose (DM) is calculated with the formula:

$$DM = \frac{\text{desired } \bar{C}_{EE}.\ CL_T.T}{F} \quad \text{(Eq. 5)}$$

Where F = availability taken from respective literature [5]. When the drug is to be administered intravenously, the rate of injection or infusion is obtained by multiplying the body clearance of the drug by the concentration desired.

To achieve greater accuracy and precision, the pharmacokinetic data used in the above equations need to be the most recent values of the patient under treatment. Unless these requisites are fulfilled, the treatment regimen will be less accurate and precise. For instance, when the pharmacokinetic data from the literature is the only information at hand, the accuracy and precision will be less.

Dose rate = CL_T. C_{EE} desired infusion. (Eq.6)

Individualization of Dose Regimen

Due to interindividual variability in pharmacokinetic of a great number of drugs, to get a better therapeutic success, individualization of the treatment regimen is required for every patient. There are examples in the literature that bring into evidence the consequences of not taking into account such variability [6-7].

Practical Example on the Way to Design or Adjust a Treatment Regimen from Pharmacokinetic Data

Case 1

Design of treatment regimen based on the pharmacokinetic data obtained from the patient. A six-month old male infant whose current weight is 7.6 kg, with a diagnosis of bacterial neuro-infection and seizure crisis was treated with ceftriaxone, DPH and dexamethasone. Metronidazole was indicated three days after suspicion of probable septicemia by anaerobic germs.

Due to possible interferences between DPH and dexamethasone on the ability of hepatic biotransformation, by enzymatic induction phenomenon [8] and with the objective of optimizing the treatment, pharmacokinetic parameters were determined to design the therapeutic regimen after the first administration of 80 mg of metronidazole by intravenous infusion for 30 minutes. The metronidazole concentrations determined at different times are shown below in Table 2.

Table 2. The metronidazole concentrations determined at different times

Time (hours)	Concentration (mcg/ml)
0.083	45.8
0.25	23.6
0.5	22.8
1.0	18.8
2.0	7.5
4.0	4.8
6.0	2.2
8.0	1.6

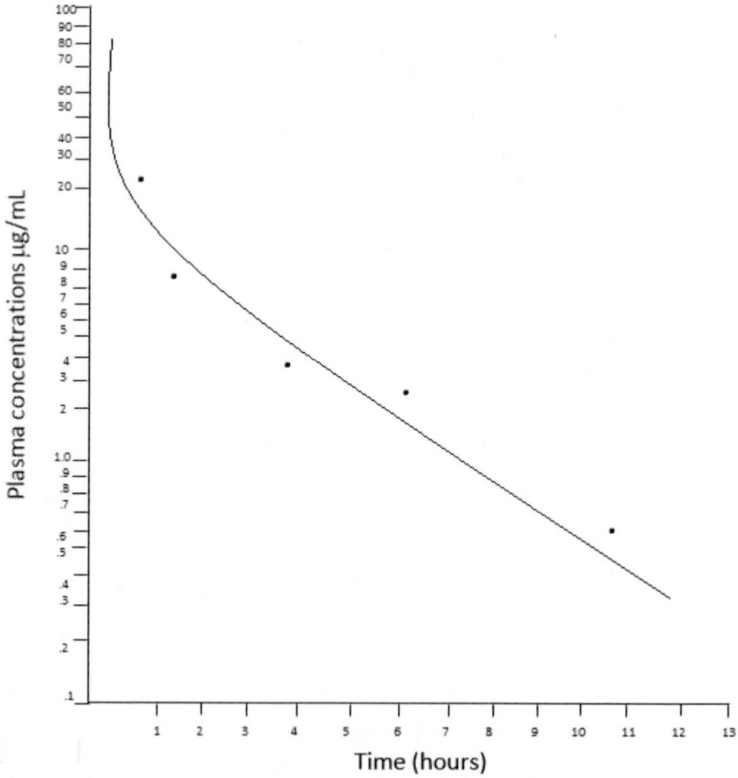

Figure 6. Decay curve of the logarithm of the plasma concentrations of an antibiotic. The points correspond to the experimental data and the curve with a continuous stripe to the data adjusted by the method of least squares.

To define the compartmental model, the curve of decay of the plasma concentrations of the drug at the different times on a semilogarithmic paper sheet is plotted (Figure 6).

This will allow us to define with certain approximation if it is an open model of one or two compartments. The example corresponds to an open model of two compartments, since two exponential phases are distinguished with the faster phase corresponding to distribution and the slower phase to elimination.

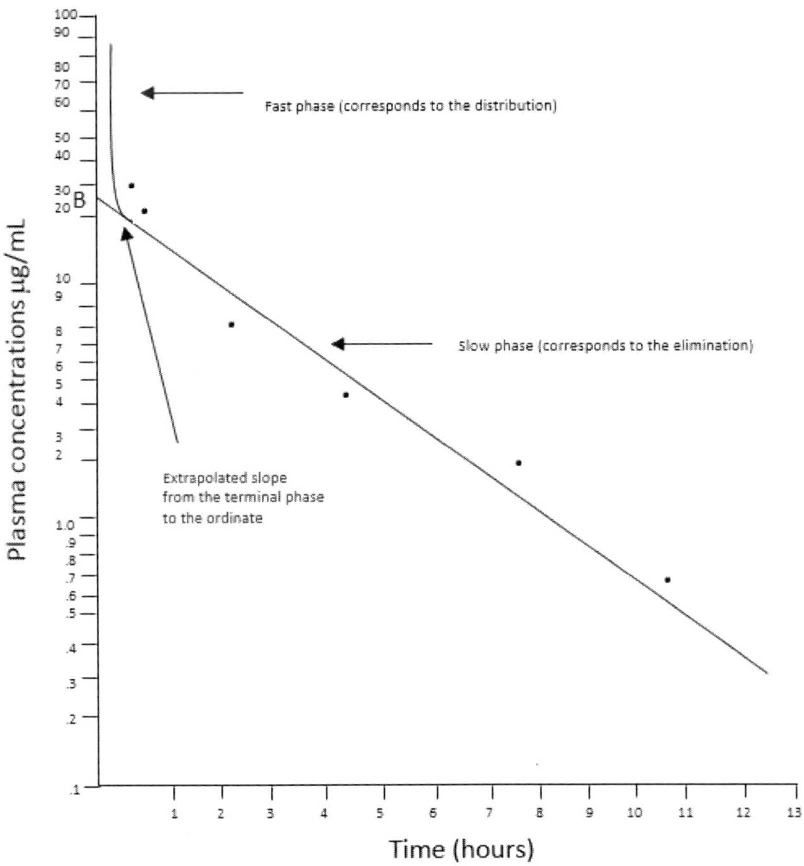

Figure 7. After obtaining the adjusted curve from the experimental data, the slow phase (elimination) is extrapolated to the ordinate, so that the alpha slope can be subsequently calculated using the residual method.

Once the number of exponential phases is defined, the extrapolated intercept is obtained at the ordinate of the terminal phase (β) and corresponds to a value of β = 22.14 μg/mL (Figure 7). To obtain the intercept of the distribution phase, the following is done: subtract the extrapolated concentrations corresponding to each time in the first phase from each of the concentrations observed in the distribution phase and the result is the slope whose intercept extrapolated to the ordinate corresponds to the value A = 65.0 mg/ml (Figure 8).

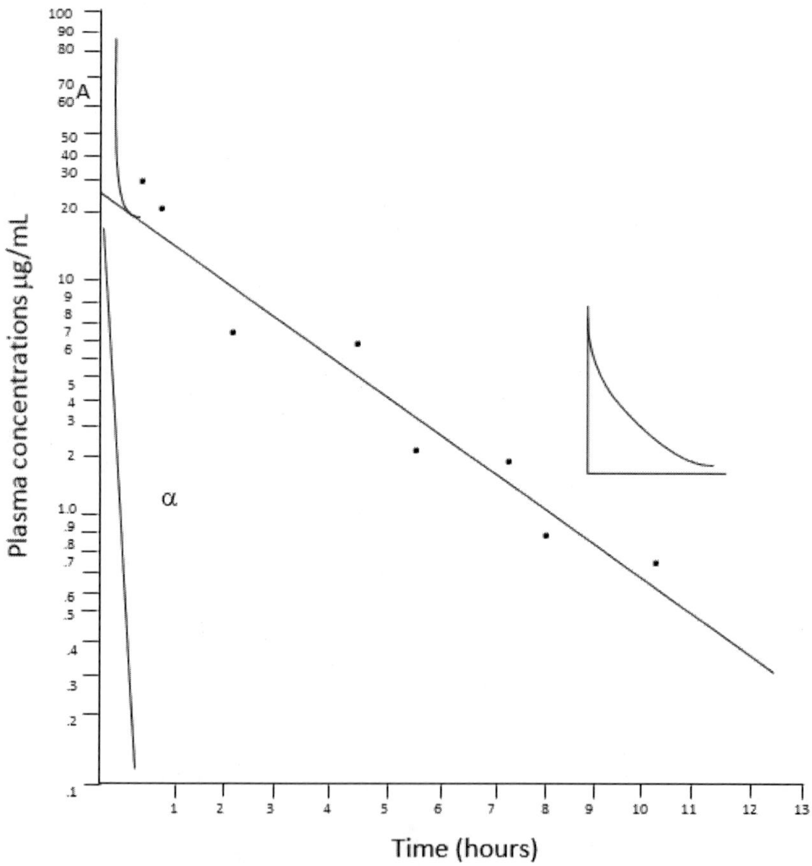

Figure 8. Residual method to obtain the value of alpha (α) slope. In the box to the right of the figure, the difference between observed and extrapolated concentrations is presented which when plotted determine the alpha slope.

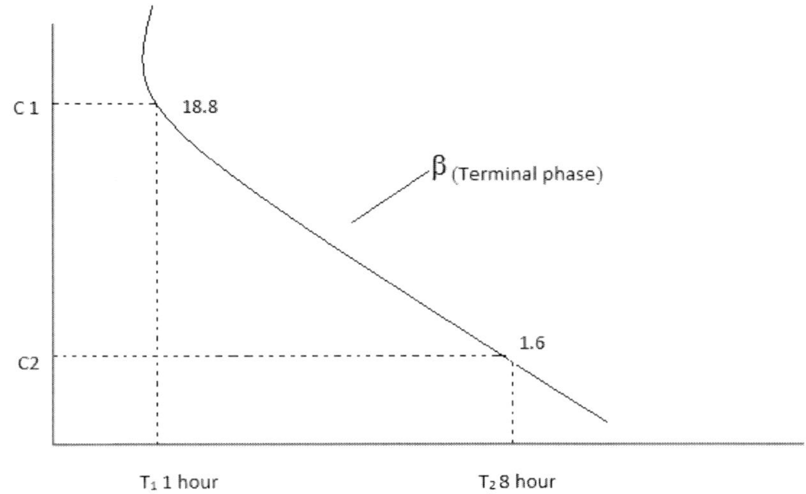

$$\beta = \frac{\text{Inc- Inc}_2}{t^2\text{-}t^1} = \frac{2.933\text{-}0.470}{8\text{-}1} = \frac{2.463}{7} = 0.3178\text{-}h^{-1}$$

Figure 9. As can be seen in the figure with only two determinations corresponding to the terminal phase (elimination) the value of the slope can be obtained which corresponds to elimination rate constant (Kel) for a mono-compartmental model.

Finally, the value of the slope of the terminal phase (β) that corresponds to the exponential data (Figure 9) and the elimination rate constant is obtained by linear regression analysis.

For that, the natural logarithm of the concentrations of such terminal phase is obtained, see Table 3:

Table 3. Natural logarithm of the concentrations of terminal phase

Time (hours)	Concentration (µg/mL)	Natural logarithm of concentration
1.0	18.8	2.933
2.0	7.5	2.014
4.0	4.8	1.568
6.0	2.2	0.788
8.0	1.6	0.470

Later the value of the slope is obtained.

$$\beta = \frac{Inc_1 - Inc_2}{t_2 - t_1} = \frac{2.933 - 0.470}{8 - 1} = \frac{2.463}{7} = 0.3518$$

Once both the values of (β) and the values corresponding to the intercepts A and B are derived, the plasma concentration at zero time (Cp^o) is the sum of these values. Thus,

$$\begin{aligned} Cp^o &= A + B \\ &= 65.05 + 22.1 \\ &= 87.19 \end{aligned}$$

From these values, the rest of the parameters required to design a treatment regimen can be calculated. Thus,

$$t1/2 = \frac{0.693}{\beta} = \frac{0.693}{0.3718} = 1.86 \text{ h}$$

$Vd = Dose = 80mg = 9.19$ L

$A+B = 8.71$ mg/mL

Dividing Vd value by body weight, we have

9.19L/7.6 kg = 1.20 L/kg

$CL_T = \beta.Vd = 0.3718\ h^{-1}$

1.2 L/kg = 0.446 L/kg/h

After obtaining the pertinent pharmacokinetic parameters to design the treatment regimen, the values obtained are substituted in the equation 7 to calculate the loading dose (LD) of the drug needed to reach the therapeutic concentration at a steady state (C_{EE}). Thus

$$LD = C_{EE} \text{ desired. } Vd \qquad \text{(Eq.7)}$$

Substituting values, we have:

LD = 15mg/L. 091 L= 13.75 mg

When the maintenance dose is known, equation 4 can be used.

To determine the loading dose through continuous intravenous infusion with the aim of maintaining the desired concentration of 15 mg/L, the equation 6 is used.

Infusion dose rate = $CL_T.C_{EE}$ desired:

= 0.3390 L/h . 15 mg/L

= 5.08 mg/h

Hence, this value will correspond to 40 mg in every 8 hours which is half of the doses administered and 120 mg in 24 hours.

Case 2

Design of a treatment regimen from pharmacokinetic data was obtained in the literature.

A 12- year-old female patient, current body weight 26.5 kg with end-stage chronic renal failure and secondary anemia who presented an infectious process requiring treatment with ampicillin, where it is intended to establish the therapeutic plan considering the pharmacokinetic of this drug.

Given the impossibility of obtaining the pharmacokinetic parameters from the same patient for lacking the analytical method to measure the plasma concentrations of the drug, the pharmacokinetic parameters were obtained from a research performed in aneurysmal children [9] to rationally design a treatment regimen. The desired plasma concentrations of ampicillin are 15 mg/L.

To calculate the loading dose, it is necessary to know the desired plasma concentrations and the volume of distribution and these were reported in a revised article with values corresponding to a median of 0.073 L/kg. The values were substituted in the formula 7 as follows:

$$LD = \bar{C}_{EE}\ \text{desired}\ .Vd\ .\text{body weight} \qquad \text{(Eq.7)}$$

$$LD = 15\ mg/L.0.073L.26.5kg = 29.0mg.$$

Subsequently, the maintenance dose (MD) is calculated using the equation 5 once the reported median value of drug clearance in the same article is obtained. Hence,

$$MD = \frac{C_{EE}\ \text{desired}\ .\ CL_T\ .\text{weight}\ .t}{F}$$

$$MD = \frac{15\ mg/L.0.003\ mL/kg/h\ .26.5\ kg \times 6\ h}{0.9} = 8.0mg/6h$$

Since it is a patient with severe renal failure, the dose corresponds to 1.0 mg/kg per day approximately.

In case of maintaining the usual dose of 50 mg/kg/day divided into four doses, each dose should be applied every two days if drug accumulation is to be avoided. The way to obtain the interval of administration should take into account the elimination half-life of the drug in the patient and in subjects without a renal problem.

The formula used to do this is as follows:

$$\text{New } T = \text{usual } T \times \frac{t1/2el \text{ of the patient}}{\text{Normal } t1/2} \qquad \text{(Eq. 8)}$$

Case 3

Adjustment of a therapeutic regimen in a patient with an established dosage plan. A 15-year-old adolescent, body weight 40 kg, without hepatic or renal dysfunction who presented salmonellosis that required treatment with oral chloramphenicol 500mg every 6hours. The treatment regimen has been applied for three days. Therefore, it is assumed that the plasma concentrations are in a steady state. In order to assess the therapeutic regimen, the concentrations before the administration of the first dose in the morning and 1.5 hours after were measured. The concentrations reported were 33.0 and 20.0 mg/L respectively. Given the risk of toxicity, it is required to adjust the dose to get a minimum concentration of 10 mg/L.

To obtain the maintenance dose, it is important to take into account the minimum desired concentration in the steady state as well as the minimum concentration found, hence the values should be substituted in the equation 9:

$$MD = \frac{\bar{C}_{EE}\text{ desired. MD used}}{\bar{C}_{EE}\text{found}} \qquad \text{(Eq.9)}$$

$$MD = \frac{10\text{ mg/L. }500\text{mg}}{20\text{ mg/L}} = \frac{5000}{20} = 250\text{ mg}$$

REFERENCES

[1] Kung HC, Huang PY, Chen WT, Ko BS, Chen YC, Chang SC, Chuang YC. 2016 guidelines for the use of antifungal agents in patients with invasive fungal diseases in Taiwan. *J Microbiol Immunol Infect* 2017. pii: S1684-1182(17)30146-9.

[2] Kantae V, Krekels EHJ, Esdonk MJV, Lindenburg P, Harms AC, Knibbe CAJ, Van der Graaf PH, Hankemeier T. Integration of pharmacometabolomics with pharmacokinetics and pharmacodynamics: towards personalized drug therapy. *Metabolomics* 2017;13:9.

[3] Colburn WA, Lee JW. Biomarkers, validation and pharmacokinetic-pharmacodynamic modelling. *Clin. Pharmacokinet* 2003;42:997-1022.

[4] Horcajada JP. Aplicabilidad de los parámetros PK/PD de losantimicrobianos en el tratamiento de infeccionescomplejas y resistenciasextremas. *Rev Esp Quimioter* 2015; 28 (Suppl. 1): 16-18. [Applicability of PK / PD parameters of antimicrobials in the treatment of complex infections and extreme resistances. *Rev Esp Quimioter* 2015; 28 (Suppl. 1): 16-18].

[5] Ritachel WA. *Handbook of basic pharmacokinetics*, 2a. Ed. Hamilton H., Drug Intelligence Publications. Inc, 1980:413-27.

[6] Zhang Z, Gu H, Zhao H, Liu Y, Fu S, Wang M, Zhou W, Xie Z, Yu H, Huang Z, Gao X. Pharmacometabolomics in endogenous drugs: a new approach for predicting the individualized pharmacokinetics of cholic acid. *J Proteome Res* 2017.

[7] Phapale PB, Kim SD, Lee HW, Lim M, Kale DD, Kim YL, Cho JH, Hwang D, Yoon YR. An integrative approach for identifying a metabolic phenotype predictive of individualized pharmacokinetics of tacrolimus. *Clin Pharmacol. Ther.* 2010;87:426-36.

[8] Chen N, Cui D, Wang Q, Wen Z, Finkelman RD, Welty D. In vitro drug-drug interactions of budesonide: inhibition and induction of transporters and cytochrome P450 enzymes. *Xenobiotica* 2017:1-10.

[9] Lares AI, Jimenez MA, Guzman A, Zaltzman S, Cravioto J. Farmacocinetica de la amplicilina en niños anéfricos siny durantehemodialisis y en sujetosnormales. *Bol Med. Hosp. Infant. Mex* 1987;44:677-84. [Pharmacokinetics of ampicillin in sinic aneurysms during hemodialysis and in normal subjects. *Bol Med. Hosp. Infant. Mex,* 1987;44:677-84].

In: The Optimization of Drug Prescribing … ISBN: 978-1-53612-263-3
Editor: Hugo Juarez Olguin

Chapter 7

THERAPEUTIC DRUG MONITORING IN CHILDREN

Hugo Juarez Olguín[1,2,*], Monica Punzo Soto[1] and Belen Juárez Tapia[1]

[1]Laboratorio de Farmacología, Instituto Nacional de Pediatría, Mexico City, Mexico

[2]Departamento de Farmacología, Facultad de Medicina, Universidad Nacional Autónoma de México, Mexico

ABSTRACT

Therapeutic drug monitoring (TDM) is an exercise that permits the pediatrician to optimize the regimens of medical treatment in an adequate form, taking into consideration the timely evaluation of the concentrations produced by the administration of a drug as a decisive indicator to adjust the number of doses of the drug and to individualize treatment based on the observed clinical responses as the need arises.

In the present report, we reviewed the most relevant clinical aspects to carry out TDM. Moreover, the most important pharmacological basis

* Corresponding Author Email: juarezol@yahoo.com

both for the interpretation of concentration values and the values required to effect dose adjustment is analyzed. Likewise, the criteria for the choice of suitable analytical method for the quantification of drug of interest were reviewed. Finally, some recommendations were directed to the physician in order to perform an adequate monitoring that contributes to the clinical-pharmacological control of their patients.

BACKGROUND

A number of retrospective and prospective studies have demonstrated the clinical utility of performing Therapeutic drug monitoring (TDM). For instance, in a three-year prospective study carried out in an epileptic patients, the monitoring of phenytoin levels and its dose adjustment based on the results of such exercise gave way to a decrease in the annual average of cases of patients with major mal seizure from figures of 5.8 before the study to 1.6 per analyzed patient after TDM [5].

In another study of the same category with ethosuximide, the number of patients whose seizure crisis was controlled ascended from 64 to 81% after carrying out TDM with its respective dose adjustment [6]. According to a more recent retrospective study, the survival rate of patients that overcome sepsis burns by gram-negative germs increased from 33 to 64% following the monitoring of gentamicin concentrations, opportune dosage corrections and individualizations [7].

Another report indicated the importance of monitoring the levels of theophylline and its respective adjustment of individual doses concluding that such activity is necessary for the control of critically ill patients [8].

Also, in an oral treatment of patients with chronic obstructive airways who were given adjusted doses, in which individual dose regimens were used to maintain adequate serum concentrations, there was an important increase in pulmonary function, corroborated by clinical test before and after TDM [8].

THERAPEUTIC DRUG MONITORING

Therapeutic drug monitoring (TDM) is one of the fundamental supportive activities for pediatric care service, because it is a key point for the physicians to achieve optimal treatment based on the therapeutic agents chosen. During TDM, the determination of serum drug concentration of the patient, obtained at the right moment and interpreted under suitable clinical and pharmacokinetic contexts, is a vital step for the individualization of dosages of many drugs [1, 3].

When analyzing the concentrations of a drug, a number of factors should be considered. The pediatric population has peculiar features and owing to their age and genetic characteristics, they possess different response behavior to drugs when compared with the adults or other individuals. Furthermore, the relation between the dose of a drug and the resulting concentrations are affected by factors as bioavailability of the dosage form used, drug therapy employed, concomitant diseases, the body weight of the patient, the distribution in different body compartments, and individual metabolic and excretion rates [1]. In recent years, clinical studies in pediatrics have shown that the doses administered in children are frequently insufficient or excessive consequently, TDM has gained a relevant importance for those who are directly involved in the therapeutic management of the patients [4].

PHARMACOLOGICAL BASIS

To efficiently carry out TDM, it is necessary to review a number of theoretical concepts that would facilitate the understanding of the basic principles of drug interactions in the organism that guarantee the achievement of the desired pharmacological effect. When the doses of a drug are administered, the maximum plasma concentration of the drug will be produced in a time range and this should be measured on finishing the distribution phase of the drug to verify if it is within the post-distribution therapeutic limit [9]. In majority of the drugs, the distribution phase occurs within an interval of 0.5 to 2 hours, although there are situations where the distribution phase is prolonged for up to 6 or 8 hours as is the case of digoxin and digitoxin respectively.

The minimum concentration is generally measured a little before the administration of the next dose and this has the objective of discovering if the plasma level of the drug is above the effective minimum concentration and if the drug is being eliminated from the organism with adequate speed.

The approximate time to reach the maximum and minimum concentrations of a drug within a dosing interval varies depending on the physiochemical properties of the drug and its different presentations. Pharmacological treatments require that the doses be repeated at a defined time, which is achieved by following a dosage regimen that stipulates the administration interval that ensures the obtention of adequate pharmacological response and sustained through a time period during which the administration of the drug at determined dose is repeated.

Any drug that enters the body is eliminated through different routes at different speeds, which depend on the half-life elimination time, defined as the time required for the plasma concentration of a drug to reduce by 50%. The half-life elimination time is a parameter that marks the main guideline in the elaboration of dosage regimens. When repeated doses of a medicine are administered at regular intervals, the levels in the serum increase until equilibrium between the administered doses and the eliminated amount of the drug is achieved. Once this phase is reached, the plasma concentration level of the medicine becomes steady; a phase regarded as a steady state. This phase is obtained after four or five half-lives of the medicine have passed [9]. Most drugs have already had their established serum concentration therapeutic ranges, defined by a minimum effective concentration and a maximum tolerated concentration.

Clinical experience has shown that for all drugs and depending on the clinical diagnosis, there is a minimum serum concentration, under which the desired pharmacological effect is usually not perceived, and maximum plasma level, above which the toxic effects may exceed the therapeutic benefit and hence, increases the occurrence and/or severity of adverse reactions or toxicity.

Relationship Dose-Concentration-Effect

As a form of control for adequate use of medicines, it has been demonstrated that the intensity of a pharmacological action for most of the drugs is more closely associated with the blood concentrations than the doses that were administered to reach the said levels. Although, it has been observed that there can be great variability in the dose-response relationship among patients, the concentration of a drug depends on the "compliance" of the patient and in the case of a child, on his/her relatives to give the child the medicine in the right dose and at the right time, as well as on the processes of absorption, distribution, biotransformation and excretion, which in turn are related to the regional blood flow, the degree of plasma protein binding and the transport mechanism of the drug to reach effective levels at the site of action. Therefore, the clinical application of drug monitoring is limited to those that demonstrate a correlation between a range of concentrations and a pharmacological effect. Given this correlation, there are a number of useful indications, as discussed below, to determine whether the plasma levels of drugs should be controlled.

Individual Variability

For the predisposition which some patients present in response to the administration of a drug, some of them can tolerate higher or lower plasma levels to obtain the desired therapeutic effects. Considering individual variability, the benefits of TDM are exemplified by the results achieved in phenytoin monitoring in a German hospital in which patients who showed any kind of renal insufficiency concomitantly treated with other anticonvulsants were pooled and monitored. The result revealed a reduction in the recommended inferior limit of phenytoin levels as well as its toxicity limit levels. At the same time, the proportion of levels within the therapeutic range values increased significantly from 38% to 64% after being pooled [10].

This information shows the importance of TDM in determining the adequate time to adjust dosage regimens and to individualize the dosage regimens since individual variability could be a result of other factors worthy of consideration that may alter the response to the drug (Figure 1).

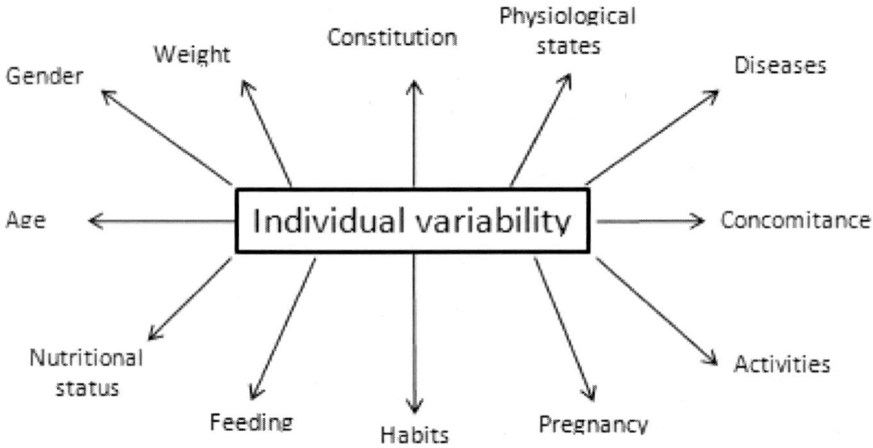

Figure 1. Factors that affect the response to a drug.

Clinical Indications for the Measurement of Drug Concentrations

In the management of patients requiring drug therapies, a number of situations in which it is necessary and sometimes urgent to perform TDM often arise. For instance, in cases where the administration of an overdose of the indicated drug are suspected or in problems where a drug not prescribed is mistakenly administered or even in situations where the desired effect are not obtained (lack of therapeutic response). The first important requisite in the measurement of drug concentrations is to count with an available analytical method to quantify the concentrations and to ensure the existence of a relationship between dose-concentration-effect for the procedures to be followed based on such relationship. Below is a list of some justifiable indications for the performance of TDM.

1) To establish the optimal dose of a drug in cases where it is not possible to measure its response, especially when there is no means or parameters to do that.
2) To carry out the monitoring of prophylactic drugs in order to detect if the effect is insufficient to maintain the prevention of the target disease and avoid its unexpected manifestation.
3) When toxicity due to high levels of drug is suspected. In such a situation, it becomes necessary to know the concentrations of the drug and the best way to treat it, especially if the symptoms are already present. An illustration of this could be the case of ventricular cardiac sounds in a premature probably due to toxicity by digitalis. However, it is essential to have the capacity to differentiate adverse drug effects owing to high level of a drug from other causes. For instance, tachycardia is not always a diagnosis of theophylline overdose, since this sign is also found in patients with severe airway obstruction.
4) To establish dose limit for a drug. To do this, it is extremely necessary to know the concentrations of the drug in certain special situations. An example is when drug interactions are suspected or when the pharmacokinetic parameters show substantial intra and interindividual variability, even when the first-step effect is present to a large degree.
5) Another indication to perform TDM is the disease state of the patients, since such conditions may alter drug absorption, protein binding, and elimination or cause the accumulation of active metabolites. Therefore, It is of paramount importance to determine the drug concentrations when changes in bioavailability is

suspected as well as when the occurrence of adverse effects is persistent, as could be seen during high-dose therapy of methotrexate where the production of adverse reactions could occur and usually this is attacked with the administration of adjusted dose of leucovorin depending on the serum concentration of methotrexate [2].

Drugs That Must Be Monitored

A number of criteria have been considered to justify and select which drugs should be monitored. Such criteria reside on a) drugs whose toxicity is very dangerous and the evolution of such toxicity is not clinically well-defined, b) drugs whose dose-response relationship is very marked, c) drugs with narrow therapeutic range that are used for long periods of treatment, d) drugs whose use is fraught with risk for the life of the patient, e) those whose pharmacokinetics present considerable interindividual variability, f) drugs that follow a nonlinear kinetic since their elimination is easily saturated, g) drugs that are widely distributed in the body and have a reliable analytic method for their determination.

In addition, other groups of drugs such as some immunosuppressants like cyclosporin A, some antibiotics, neuroleptics, and certain antidepressants have been included even when the concentration limits of some of them are still under investigation. Due to the great progress made in terms of analytical technology, the number of drugs that are incorporated into TDM process is increasing [11].

Procedure for TDM

To carry out TDM, it is important to follow a series of activities which begins with filling out the format for the study in a correct and complete form. Such format is previously designed in such a way that it contains all the necessary information required for a good performance of the monitoring not only for the medical staff but also for the person that requires it. The data that must be included in the request are as follows: a) General date: patient´s name, the clinical file number or code, age, sex, weight, height, gestational age, heart rate, temperature, diagnosis and the present clinical status; b) Drug to monitor: generic name of the drug, manufacturer, lot number and pharmaceutical presentation although, they are not strictly necessary; c) Drug doses: impregnation or maintenance dose, treatment onset, present dose - time and route of administration; and d) Clinical data: manifestation of toxicity, simultaneous drugs, metabolic alkalosis or acidosis, urea, creatinine, total bilirubin and total proteins.

Generally, on the reverse of the request form, the recommendations for a sample taken (schedule and conditions) are written and usually this part contains a blank space for the report on the studies, observations and suggestions.

Timely Sampling for Drug Monitoring

Punctuality in the administration of the drug and blood sample collection at the indicated schedules is vital for correct interpretation of the concentrations during TDM.

The opportune time for sampling is mainly based on the pharmaceutical presentation used and the administration route as well as the pharmacokinetic characteristics and other previously mentioned urgent reasons for the sample test.

In addition, to make a correct interpretation of the results, it is necessary to know the time that has elapsed since the last administration of the drug including if this has prolonged beyond the indicated dose range. For TDM to be useful, samples should be preferably taken until the steady state is reached, as there is a previous drug accumulation process that is in agreement with the elimination half-life of the drug.

When a treatment is started at a constant dose, the steady state is reached in a lapse of at least five half-life of the drug which corresponds to the time when 97% of the concentrations, referred to as the equilibrium state, is reached [9] (Figure 2).

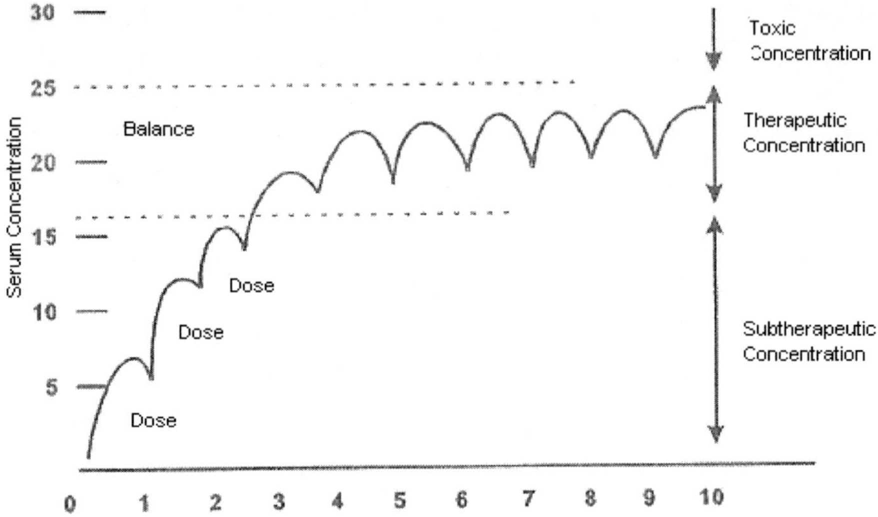

Figure 2. Relationship between the half-life of a drug and the steady state.

For compounds like phenytoin or phenobarbital, the time when blood sample should be taken is generally not definitive because the difference between the minimum and maximum concentrations on reaching the steady state is very small. In other kinds of drugs like theophylline, aminoglycosides and other antiarrhythmics with narrow therapeutic range and relatively short half-life, it is advisable to take the blood samples in a timely manner with the objective of establishing if the choice of the dose is adequate due to its rapid elimination [12].

Analytical Method

To carry out TDM, it is an indispensable requisite to count on an available analytical method for its quantification. The development of new analytical techniques has made it possible to practically quantify the vast majority of drugs in all kinds of biological fluid like serum, plasma, blood, urine, amniotic liquid, gastric juice, biliary secretion, etc., when there are trained and qualified personnel for taking samples of these fluids and consider the ethical and clinical aspects to decide on taking such samples. Once the samples are taken with the recommendations and in the indicated schedule, the best method for its quantification should be chosen. The choice of this depends on a number of criteria which are listed and discussed below.

Reliability: The chosen method should be reliable. This means that it must prove to be reproducible, sensitive, specific, exact and precise during its validation process. Each of these parameters has its error variations based on statistical test giving validity to the same.

Demand: When a quantification method is thought to be used for the monitoring service, the demand which such method has should be considered. This is because this point constitutes one of the principal factors to decide on whether to use it or not. For example, a method of atomic absorption is limited to measuring only a few compounds and hence, its acquisition and maintenance is costly for the hospital.

Sample amount: One important characteristic to perform TDM is the sample volume necessary for processing and quantifying the drug of interest. Sometimes, it is difficult to take a big volume of blood especially in pediatric patients particularly in those with some level of undernourishment or in the cases of a newborn whose body fluid may be decompensated by taking samples. In the face of this situation, new methods like the immunoenzymatics that require a minimum volume of blood (approximately 10 microliters) have been developed. The advantage of this rotates on the fact that it does not require the extraction of the compound to carry out the measurement of the substance.

Time of analysis: In the vast majority of the cases, like those where an intoxication produced by an overdose of a drug is suspected, it is required to obtain the result as soon as possible because of the clinical situation of the patient. On the other hand, there are methods whose result may last a little longer and such methods are principally assigned for research projects, where the results are not required urgently.

Among the methods that stand out for their speed to obtain results is enzyme-linked immunosorbent assay (ELISA) which is based on instant reaction between an antigen (drug) and antibody in a wide range of concentrations. However, few methods such as high-performance liquid chromatography (HPLC) results are versatile and it is based on a separation of the drug between two phases by physicochemical affinity, detection and quantification in relation to an increased response factor. This method is applied to quantify the vast majority of drugs used in the hospitals. Table 1 shows a comparison between ELISA and HPLC (analytical methods most used to perform TDM) which outlines the advantages and disadvantages of each according to the evaluation criteria previously cited.

Table 1. Comparison of analytical methods used in drug monitoring

Characteristics	AIA (ELISA)	HPLC
Time of analysis	2 - 3 minutes	25 minutes
Requires extraction	Not	Yes
Dependable	Yes	Yes
Sensitive	Yes	Yes
Use of reagents:		
Expiration	Short	Long
Contamination	Yes	Not
Cost per determination	6 - 7 USD	1.5 USD
Needs medical staff	Not	Yes

EIA = Enzyme immunoassay test.
HPLC = High performance liquid chromatography.

Interpretation of Results

The serum concentrations of a drug should be interpreted under a clinical setting taking into account the information contained in the application. The therapeutic intervals have been established based on clinical studies with the intention of giving interpretations in which both factors must be related (concentration-effect). Such levels could be reported with different values however, they should be handled with care and only as a general guide.

The results obtained in a TDM study must be interpreted in accordance with the clinical situation of the patient using the data included in the application. When a value outside the therapeutic range is obtained, a precise review of the information in the format should be made before making the dose adjustments [1]. It has been seen that there are other factors that can alter the effect which drug concentration could produce at the site of action. For example, a concentration of digoxin which is therapeutic for the majority of the patients may be excessive for a patient with hypokalemia, hypercalcemia, acid-base disorder, hypoxemia or with advanced coronary artery disease. Occasionally, the patients show an adequate therapeutic effect even when they are in a subtherapeutic drug concentration or in potentially toxic levels [13].

Another factor in interpreting drug concentration results is the ability of such drug to bind plasma proteins, although at different degrees. For instance, phenytoin binds at a degree of approximately 92% to proteins. It has been found that the concentration of unbound drug to protein will correspond more closely to the amount of the drug at the receptor site. Therefore, the determination of total drug concentration could be misinterpreted, especially if the percentage of the drug binding to protein will, for various causes, be significantly modified and thus, the fraction of free drug. With regard to this point, the nutritional status of pediatric patients is a factor that must be carefully taken into account, since an alteration in the protein levels directly affects the fraction of the free drug and their manifestations. Likewise, as important as the above, factors such as interactions among drugs having an affinity with the proteins; uremia involved cases; renal or hepatic insufficiency and variations in protein levels especially albumin (or gamma globulins for other drugs) can alter protein binding process [14].

As a way bellying up to the real concentration of a drug, a number of techniques to determine the free fraction have been proposed.

Ultrafiltration has been the most used method to determine this fraction, especially for the advantages which it has over other methods like dialysis, ultra centrifugation and gel filtration [15].

Dose Adjustment

Some patients can develop tolerance to certain drugs, especially when they are used for a prolonged period. In such cases, the upper therapeutic concentration limit may increase. Moreover, it has been found that the doses of some drugs need to be modified or adjusted when they are administered together with other drugs with either synergic or antagonistic action. For example, in newborns a serum concentration of phenytoin that is considered "within the therapeutic range" may produce symptoms of toxicity when simultaneously administered with phenobarbital [16-18]. In addition, the existence of pharmacologically active metabolites as well as the changes that may occur at the level of protein binding should also be taken into account at the time of making dose adjustment. Among the factors that can cause certain alterations in the expected levels in patients are: noncompliance of the patient, administration of inadequate dose, bad absorption, low bioavailability of the preparation, drug interactions. Renal or hepatic insufficiency, protein binding alteration and slow or fast metabolism owing to genetic factors [19]. In case of finding any factor present, it is appropriate to make dose adjustment.

For the case of drugs that follow a linear kinetic, the most common model to make this adjustment is as follows:

New dose = Previous dose x (Desired concentration / Previous concentration)

Whenever a change in dosage is made, it is necessary to carry out TDM again in the steady state so as to verify if the change in dosage produced the expected concentration [9].

Dosage Regimen

To establish a dosage regimen that would produce an adequate pharmacological response, there are two adjustment parameters that can be estimated according to the pharmacological parameters. Such adjustment parameters are a) dosage interval or time interval in which the administration of a drug is repeated and b) dose, defined as the amount of drug administered in order to get a determined effect. These parameters can be estimated from the pharmacokinetic profile as elimination half-life, the volume of distribution and clearance, etc.

In addition, there are three methods to establish dosage regimen.

Empirical Method

This method is based only on the clinical response of the patient. For example, if manifestations of toxicity are observed, the drug is either suspended or the dose is reduced, while the existence of unsatisfactory pharmacological response demands an increase in dose as deemed necessary.

Pharmacokinetic Method

This method is applied based on the calculation of some pharmacokinetic parameters using mathematical models for calculating the best dosage regimen and in this way individualize the treatment on the basis of specific characteristics of the patient. Many authors have developed monograms to facilitate the calculation of the pharmacokinetic parameters and in this manner are able to use reported mathematical models to establish dosage regimen.

Drug Monitoring Method

This procedure is based on the knowledge of the concentrations of a drug at fixed times (corresponding to its minimum and maximum concentrations in steady state) and it is always supported by clinical observations. It is suggested that this method should be used simultaneously with pharmacokinetic procedure in order to establish in a precise form the dosage regimen.

Observations and Recommendations for TDM

One of the most important activities during the process of TDM is its report. This should include both the results of the levels of the samples analyzed and their interpretations. Depending on the concentrations reached, the levels could be classified as therapeutic, subtherapeutic or toxic determined with reference to the therapeutic range reported in the literature.

Furthermore, additional comments on the result which was derive from the clinical status of the patient can be added to the report. For example, when there is any alteration in the concentration, it affect the relationship that is surely caused by individual variability factor.

As already mentioned, it is sometimes possible to calculate some pharmacokinetic parameters including the absorption and elimination profiles or both and with them, individualized dose adjustment can be made for the patient [20].

It has also been demonstrated that this last step of monitoring would be more effective if the results and the recommendations accompanying the study report are adequately and timely elaborated. Nevertheless, it would not be possible if the application is incompletely filled especially when this is on necessary information that may facilitate the making of pertinent suggestions and recommendations.

In addition, evidence has also shown that the final stage of monitoring is more effective when the results and recommendations are discussed personally with the treating physicians because, in a certain way, this would guarantee compliance with the recommendations.

As a complementary part of TDM, there must be a follow-up of the studies especially when adjustment of dosage regimen was recommended together with indication to determine the concentration levels reached after a time lapse following drug adjustment or when after an evaluation of the clinical status of the patient, it was indicated or recommended to continue with the same dose. In this way, during the follow-up, it will be possible to determine if the proposed recommendations were adequate to achieve the recommended therapeutic levels as well as a means to evaluate the dose adjustment method used.

Assessment of TDM Cost-Benefit

Healthcare cost has considerably increased since the last decade. Simultaneously, the introduction of new technologies, diagnostic procedures, methods of prevention and treatment of diseases has witnessed an astronomical increase. Nevertheless, in countries like Mexico, the majority of the hospital centers including the tertiary hospitals is still in the skepticism or believes that they are outside the budget possibilities.

At present, the cost-benefit of the new techniques used in healthcare is continuously subjected to evaluation and TDM is not an exception. Therefore, before introducing any TDM technique in a hospital, it is pertinent to meditate on the cost-benefit guided by certain questions as for whether "it is beneficial to all the patients receiving therapies with a drug? Is there a correlation between the concentrations of the drug and the therapeutic effect? Is the method expensive? And what are its limitations?

TDM is an instrument of control that serves as a support for the management of drugs administrated to patients, especially the pediatric population which is an age with peculiar characteristics, however, it is not decisive [20-21]. In addition, it should not necessarily be used in all patients since it implies an expenditure of human and economic resources. Therefore, the arbitrary and unjustified use of it may slack down its benefits both for the physician and his patients [4].

TDM has been reported as fundamental for the use of aminoglycosides since in this way, it has been possible to establish the therapeutic and toxic levels of this group of drugs reported as having high individual variability [22]. In infection cases, like in severe pneumonia by gram-negative pathogens, in which the life of the patient is at risk, the treatment has been satisfactorily carried out by adjusting individual doses in relation to the elimination rates. In this way, it has been discovered that with individual doses, some patients have needed from five to six times the recommended regimen to obtain the therapeutic serum concentrations. In a retrospective study with gentamicin in which the cost-benefit was analyzed, the price, equipment maintenance cost, disposable medical accessories, salary of personnel, minor equipment and scientific journals were included. The benefits derived from TDM in the study were a reduction in mortality associated with septicemia by gram-negative pathogens, an economic increase associated with decreased mortality as well as an average cost-benefit ratio of 8.7 to 10. The authors pointed out that this type of study could be applied by any institution to find out if TDM is economically convenient and decides if it will be incorporated as a service within the hospital or in collaborations with several services since it does not only provide economic benefits but also important in improving or increasing the quality of care to the patient [21].

In a similar study in children, the benefits of TDM in an individualized therapy with theophylline were analyzed with the findings of a number of clinical advantages notably in the reduction of adverse reactions, a short stay in the wards of intensive care unit and short periods of time to begin oral therapy. This study was carried out comparing a similar group of patients to whom the dosing of theophylline was empirically assigned. The authors concluded that the application of clinical pharmacokinetics through TDM offers substantial benefits over those that are only empirical.

Adverse Effects

Majority of the drugs can produce adverse effects in the patients for the simple reason that their consumption is witnessing an increasing tendency and in occasions, it is used indiscriminately and thus, the occurrence of adverse effects with greater frequency [22]. Between 1.7% and 4.5% of hospital admissions are due to adverse reactions to drugs [23]. This has aroused the concern to create pharmacovigilance programs to timely prevent and manage drug adverse effects. In 1937, death due to renal insufficiency was registered in 76 people who took sulfanilamide elixir containing diethylene glycol. The need to create a strict and reliable laboratory for clinical tests that guarantee the safety and health of the patients had antecedent the tragedy that occurred with the use of thalidomide in pregnant women. This event was the precursor of the establishment of the committee on drug safety [24]. This committee receives reports from physicians, other professionals in health and pharmaceutical companies on all suspicions of adverse drug reactions in the post-marketing stage. Such information is integrated into a data bank. In the European Community, pharmacovigilance has been a convenient and effective procedure since 1992 [25].

In the light of the above, there is also a great concern to create pharmacovigilance program that covers the vigilance of several adverse reactions for the administration of other drugs as well as new manifestations that arise with the pharmacological doses used in patients which until date are unreported [26-27].

DISCUSSION

The decision to incorporate into the hospital environment drug monitoring service as an activity geared towards aiding clinical pharmacological control, is firstly, a fully justified procedure based on its benefits which have officially been established in various countries and little by little, other hospital institutions are incorporating it. Nevertheless, the work has not been easy for the fact that it demands infrastructure and technical resources like manpower to carry out its functions.

In terms of the first function, there are a great number of laboratory methods that could be applied in TDM, which go from immunoenzymatics methods (which even with its high cost for every determination, do not cease from being profitable on evaluating the cost-benefit) to chromatographic methods (which require the existence of technical people as well as pharmacists with a wide clinical perspective and who are in close collaboration with the treating physicians). Only these could serve as a means to propose the best treatment adjustment when necessary, with the objective of optimizing dosage regimen in an individualized form, considering the various factors which could give rise to biological variability of each patient as well as providing the needed training for considering the possible alterations in the response produced by a concentration or dose at the time of interpretation.

The establishment of pharmacovigilance centers would permit a better and greater development of medical doctors, paramedical doctors and clinical pharmacists. Therefore, it is necessary that all health professionals join hands together in a bid to create committees to support this program and form true pharmacovigilance centers that would optimally contribute to improve the health of the population.

REFERENCES

[1] Ji S, Zeng Y, Wu P, Lee EJ. Sampling schedule design towards optimal drug monitoring for individualizing therapy. *Comput Methods Programs Biomed.* 2005; 80:57-63.

[2] Oellerich M. Therapeutic drug monitoring and pharmacokinetic dose prediction methods. *Wien Klin Wochenschr Suppl.* 1992; 191:12-5.

[3] Fox BI, Felkey BG. Hospital participation in prescription drug monitoring programs. *Hosp Pharm.* 2017; 52:316-318.

[4] Fayet Mello A, Buclin T, Decosterd LA, Delhumeau C, di Iulio J, Fleurent A, Schneider MP, Cavassini M, Telenti A, Hirschel B, Calmy A. Successful efavirenz dose reduction guided by therapeutic drug monitoring. *Antivir Ther.* 2011; 16:189-97.

[5] Krasowski MD, Penrod LE. Clinical decision support of therapeutic drug monitoring of phenytoin: measured versus adjusted phenytoin plasma concentrations. *BMC Med Inform Decis Mak.* 2012; 14;12:7.

[6] Capovilla G, Beccaria F, Veggiotti P, Rubboli G, Meletti S, Tassinari CA. Ethosuximide is effective in the treatment of epileptic negative

myoclonus in childhood partial epilepsy. *J Child Neurol.* 1999; 14:395-400.

[7] Llanos-Paez CC, Staatz CE, Lawson R, Hennig S. A population pharmacokinetic model of gentamicin in pediatric oncology patients to facilitate personalized dosing. *Antimicrob Agents Chemother.* 2017; May 22. pii: AAC.00205-17.

[8] Dager Ew, Albertson ETT. Impact of therapeutic drug monitoring of intravenous theophylline regimens on serum theophylline concentrations in the medial intensive care unit. *Ann Pharmacother* 1992; 26:1287-91.

[9] Gibaldi M, Pierre D. *Pharmacokinetics*, 2a, ed. New York: Marcel Dekker, 1975.

[10] Gibaldi M. Revisiting some factors contributing to variability. *Ann Pharmacother* 1992; 26:1002-7.

[11] Staatz CE, Taylor PJ, Tett SE. Comparison of an ELISA and an LC/MS/MS method for measuring tacrolimus concentrations and making dosage decisions in transplant recipients. *Ther Drug Monit.* 2002; 24:607-15.

[12] Taylos WJ, Robinson JD, Slaughter RL. Establishing a pharmacy based therapeutic drug monitoring service. *Drug Intell Clin Pharm* 1985; 19: 818-24.

[13] Zhao L, Yang P, Li P, Wang X, Qin W, Zhang X. Efficiency of individual dosage of digoxin with calculated concentration. *Clin Interv Aging.* 2014; 9:1205-10.

[14] Yau JC, Brunner LJ, Lopez-Berenstein G, Le Maistre CF, Luke DR. Therapeutic drug monitoring of ciclosporine-lipoprotein levels. *Pharmacotherapy* 1991; 11: 291-5.

[15] Kimura S, Iyama S, Yamaguchi Y, Kanakura Y. Homogenous enzyme immunoassay for cyclosporine in whole blood using the EMIT 2000 cyclosporine specific assay with the COBAS MIRA-plus analyzer. *J Clin Lab Anal* 2001; 15:319-23.

[16] Hayes G, Kootsikas EM. Reassessing the lower end of the phenytoin therapeutic range: a review of the literature. *Ann Pharmacother* 1993; 27:1389-92.

[17] Pathak G, Upadhyay A, Pathak U, Chawla D, Goel SP. Phenobarbitone versus phenytoin for treatment of neonatal seizures: an open-label randomized controlled trial. *Indian Pediatr* 2013; 50:753-7.
[18] Bourgeois BF. Pharmacologic intervention and treatment of childhood seizure disorders: relative efficacy and safety of antiepileptic drugs. *Epilepsia* 1994; 35 Suppl 2:S18-23.
[19] Werner M. Metabolism and pharmacokinetic of aminophenazone in a man of different age and under various pathological conditions. *Agents Actions* 1982; 10: 99-107.
[20] Lippi G, Salvagno GL, Brocco G, Guidi GC. Appropriateness of theophylline plasma levels. *Arch Pathol Lab Med* 2007; 131:1166.
[21] Effting C, de Moraes Arantes A, Queiroz Labre LV, Carneiro WJ, de Oliveira Neto JR, Bariani C, Rodrigues CR, Rodrigues AR, Cunha LC. Individualizing oral busulfan dose after using a test dose in patients undergoing hematopoietic stem cell transplantation: pharmacokinetic characterization. *Ther Drug Monit.* 2015; 37:66-70.
[22] Guy C, Blay N, Rousset H, Fardeau V, Ollaguier M. Centre Regional de Pharmacovigilance, Hospital de Bellevue Saint-Etienne. *Therapie* 1990; 45: 429-31.
[23] Pere JC, Haramburu F, Salame G, Chasliere A, Diekakou H, Pelletier A, Dllams N, Begaud B. Centre de Pharmacovigilance Bordeauz-Aquitaine, Hospital Pellegrin. *Therapie* 1990; 5; 391-17.
[24] Barbadoro E. The international system of drug control. *Bull Chim Farm* 1990: 129:140-3.
[25] Begaud B, Chasliere A, Haramburu F. Organization and results of drug vigilance in France. *Rev Epidemil Santé Publique* 1994; 42: 416-23.
[26] Miremont G, Haramburu F, Begaud B, Pere JC, Dangoumau J. Adverse drug reaction: Physicians opinion versus causality assessment method. *Eur J Clin Pharmaol* 1994; 46:285-9.
[27] Flether AP. An appraisal of spontaneous adverse event monitoring. *Adverse Drug React Toxicol Rev* 1992; 114: 213-27.

In: The Optimization of Drug Prescribing … ISBN: 978-1-53612-263-3
Editor: Hugo Juarez Olguin

Chapter 8

NUTRITION AND PHARMACOKINETICS OF MEDICINES

***Ismael Lares-Asseff*[1,*], *Mayra Santillán García*[2] *and Belen Juarez Tapia*[2]**

[1]Centro de Investigación Interdisciplinario para el Desarrollo Integral Regional, Instituto Politécnico Nacional, Durango, Mexico
[2]Laboratorio de Farmacología, Instituto Nacional de Pediatría, Mexico City, Mexico

ABSTRACT

Caloric-protein severe malnutrition is a condition in which many nutritional deficiencies simultaneously occur, constituting a public health problem and, in practice, explains the high morbidity and mortality rates in the population of children, especially in developing countries. Approximately one-half of the total population of the world is estimated to have suffered and survived a period of moderate or advanced malnutrition during childhood.

It is estimated that about 1000 million children under the age of 15 years who lived in 1980, about 400 million did not receive an adequate

* Corresponding Author Email: ismaelares@yahoo.com

diet, because in their societies the same factors that interfere with the correct distribution of available foods prevailed. Due to the effect of malnutrition on the pharmacokinetics of drugs analyzed in this chapter, it is advisable to individualize the therapeutic regimens, to optimize its therapeutic management in pediatric patients principally in those who are under severe malnutrition.

BACKGROUND

The number of cases of severe caloric-protein malnutrition in relation to the high-risk population in a given period is unknown. Nevertheless, estimates in different pre-industrialized regions range from 0.5 to 7% in children under 5 years of age. According to surveys conducted in Mexico, it is estimated that in children less than 4 years of age, only 22% of those living in rural areas and 40% of those living in urban areas have normal weight.

In rural areas, 49% have first-grade malnutrition; 25%, second-grade and 2.5%, third-grade. In urban areas, the percentages are 42, 15 and 0.8% respectively [1].

Studies on infant and pre-school mortality in Latin American countries reveal that malnutrition is a direct or indirect cause of more than one-third of the deaths in children aged 0-5 years [2]. In Mexico, depending on the geographical area, the mortality rates in children less than 1 year old are 5-15 times higher than those prevalent in areas where children are in optimal health, while the mortality rates of children aged 1-4 years are 10 to 30 times higher, also considering the same geographical conditions [3].

The set of clinical and biochemical symptoms and signs that are observed in children with poor food intake (malnourishment), which at times are managed by the use of diets of varied content and low protein content is known by the name caloric-protein malnutrition. Nutritional deficiency occurs when the cells of the organism do not reckon with sufficient amount of essential nutrients to fulfill the normal metabolic functions.

PATHOGENY

Regardless of the etiology of under nutrition, its pathogenic process is essentially the mimic of a negative balance of the food nutrients. Calorigenic, plastic or regulatory nutrients have a metabolism characterized by being harmonious and supportive to the body. Thanks to the ability of the body tissues to transform chemical energy to metabolic energy, the realization of the cellular work that characterizes life in its multiple expressions is possible. In the pediatric field, a very important part of the work is referred to the functions of growth and development [4].

In malnutrition there are many different circumstances that can destroy the harmonic proportional relations between the components of the diet. Sometimes this is complete and balanced in its components, but insufficient in its energy supply. If in these cases, the constitutional momentum of growth is not slowed, the patient will continue to grow at the expense of his own proteins, especially of the muscle.

In other occasions, the child will use dietary proteins as an energy vehicle rather than as a plastic element and the result will be a secondary protein deficit, which will impede growth.

All of the above confirms that the nutritional functions are "harmonic and mutually supportive" [5], and this explains the enormous variety of clinical pictures that can cover the condition, depending on the balance that is established at a given time between requirement and nutrient supply. It should be remembered that there are a number of collateral metabolic changes that can come into play at any given time. Thus, the clinical expression of the deficiency is non-specific, but it is conditioned to the priorities of requirements, and therefore varies according to the patient's age, the tissue considered and the previous state of nutrition. The use of nutrients seems to be subject to the hierarchy or priority of functions. According to the biochemical, metabolic or functional urgency, certain tissues seem to be preserved for a longer time due to malnutrition. These urgencies would constitute the expression of homeostatic mechanisms of varying intensity and duration.

While most of the tissues of the chronic malnourished organism tend to atrophy, nerve tissue, adrenal glands or skeleton does not show this tendency. It is likely that in addition to overall growth, it is the skin and its accessory structures that first show the impact of the negative balance and along with them is the increase in the water content of the muscles as well as decrease their tonicity. However, the same does not happen with the muscles of the heart. The hematopoietic tissues are also not affected very early in uncomplicated malnutrition, and thus, in the chronically malnourished preschooler, hypervolemic, normocytic and normochromic malnutrition is the rule with the exception being spinal hypoplasia.

Nutritional neutropenia seems to be a new example of this functional hierarchy, which determines the priority in the satisfaction of the requirements. Thus, the pathogenic processes of malnutrition can be characterized by the following stages [6]:

Negative Balance

It basically corresponds to an acute period that brings about immediate homeostasis which results in a balance that can be regarded as "disharmony" in relation to the patterns considered as normal. The loss of weight, the phenomena of dilution and atrophy of the muscular masses, etc., illustrate this situation.

Detention of Growth and Development

It is already seen clinically in the subacute stage of the process. It is the expression of immediate homeostasis and can be interpreted as a tendency to maintain the previously achieved biochemical, functional and anatomical harmony. Within this group, the following phenomena are cataloged: Size growth detention, bone development and neuromotor behavior detention, and delay in the initiation of pubertal phenomena [7].

Adaptation

This is interpreted in the same sense that Selye considered the term which he alludes the meaning of chronicity, hence we can talk of late homeostasis. In this situation, the following phenomena are involved: Atrophic skin, hair loss, Cushing facies, low metabolism, decreased body temperature, normocytic and normochromic anemia, elevated gamma-globulin and perhaps, some neurotic behavioral aspects [8].

Homeorresis

When the etiological factors continue to act moderately intense that a new and final balance is not established in late homeostasis, the weight is in agreement with the size and from that moment, the physical growth will be in accordance with the somatic level reached. The balance, thus achieved at the expense of low stature is fundamental in the survival of the undernourished, which has not been given due attention.

Because of the importance of this new balance, Ramos Galván and Perez Ortiz [9], thought it prudent to give it the name of homeorresis (to reach a new equilibrium) to differentiate it from homeostasis (maintaining a previous equilibrium). The malnourished can achieve homeorresis at any time, once the subject has passed from immediate to late homeostasis and the sooner he achieves it, the better the prognosis of his function and the less the final damage in his physical growth. Gradually, data are collected to characterize biochemically and enzymatically the subject in homeorresis situation, but clinical experience seems to show that in the malnourished groups there are three moments of life in which the phenomenon occurs most frequently: at birth, at the end of the preschool age and onset of puberty.

In each of these stages, the pathogenic process described above shows that the malnourished is born exactly like the normal child of the same biological age. Depending on the achievements in physical and functional development, the experience of malnutrition provokes biochemical and other impacts that definitely fall outside what could be called "normal" for any age, and that is because the etiological factors trigger a new equilibrium, which makes the life of the malnourished possible. Waterloo shares these views by stating that "the child with chronic protein deficiency is, of course, very small and perhaps only half the weight that would correspond to his age" [10]. It is also different from the normal child in its general composition, but more important is the fact that the distribution of body proteins is altered in the malnourished. In the literature, facts demonstrating the dynamic alteration in the protein pattern of the undernourished abound.

The conclusion which can be derived from the above reflections is as follows: in chronic malnutrition there is an alteration of the protein pattern of the organism and that the distribution pattern is not static, but varies according to the intensity and duration of the protein deficiency and the energy intake. It is evident that all these phenomena bring about and lead to a change in chemical composition, functional modifications and morphological alterations in such a way that Jolliffe has summarized his known scheme (Figure 1) and the same phenomena are considered when he pointed out that the pathology of chronic malnutrition is characterized by: dilution, changes in function and atrophy [11].

According to the rate at which the phenomena mentioned above evolve, malnutrition may be acute, subacute or chronic. In practice, mixed malnutrition is the most frequent form of presentation. Whatever is the cause, inadequate nutrition leads to tissue depletion of energy reserves or autophagy, which is the crucial event in the ailment. The body has its own fat and muscle mass that are inevitably accompanied by biochemical changes. If catabolism persists, there will be functional modifications that can damage anatomical structures [12]. The pathophysiological processes of severe caloric-protein malnutrition are characterized by systematic alterations that are manifested by changes in the body composition with biochemical alterations, and hence provoke functional disorders that finally end in the alterations of the structures, which may be subject to irreversible changes.

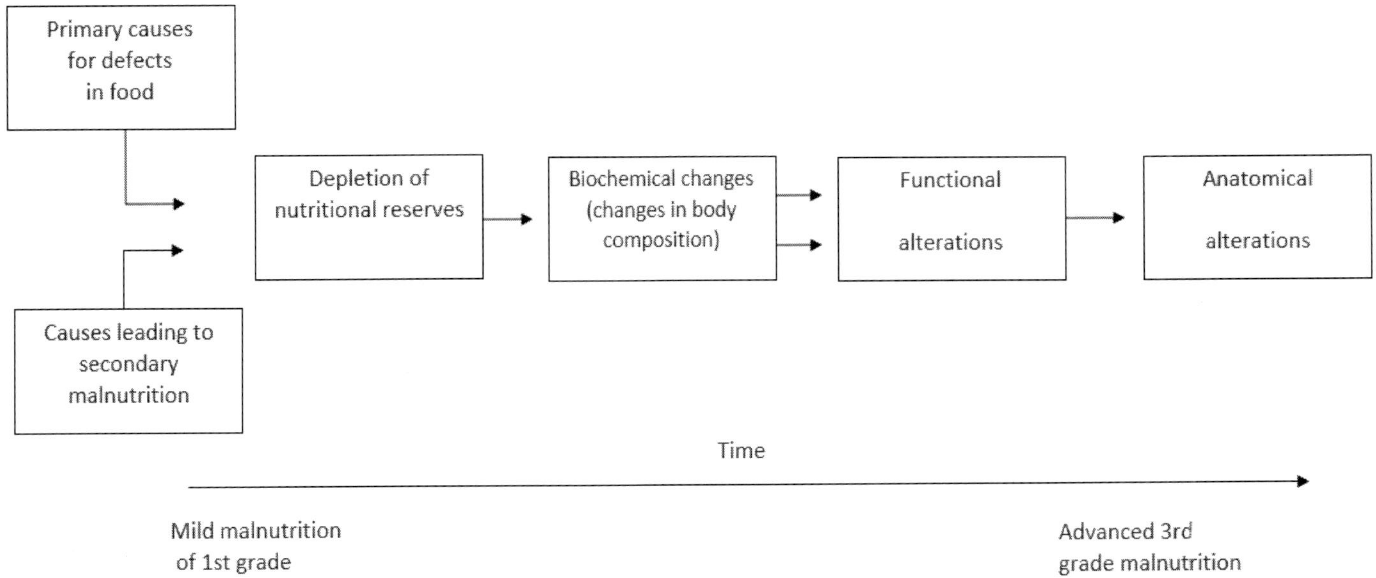

Figure 1. Pathogenesis of malnutrition. Jolliffe scheme.

This sequence of events is observed in cases where the triggering factors have persisted for a long time or of such intensity that they make the organism to rapidly pass from one stage to another. In general, the stages are not clearly separated since they overlap each other, and death may occur at any time through an inter-occurring episode of infectious type or water-electrolyte imbalance. Different organs and tissues suffer the consequences of malnutrition at different times and speed, apparently related to the position of their functional and anatomical hierarchy in the organism [13].

Severe caloric-protein malnutrition leads to a reduction in the immunological capacity, making the sufferer more vulnerable to infectious processes, thus predisposing him to concomitant diseases that require the therapeutic use of medicines.

Pathology

General Considerations

In a schematic way, the pathology of malnutrition can be summarized in two phenomena: dilution and atrophy. Modifications are added to the function, which in most cases do not represent "dysfunction" but mechanisms of homeostasis put in place by a body deprived of nutrients (Figure 2).

The obvious demonstration of these alterations consists in the chemical analysis of the child's organism as a whole, which is, in some way, beyond the scope and philosophy of the pediatrics. However, in the medical literature, the earliest descriptions of the chemical anatomy of the malnourished date back to the early twentieth century and are owed to the works of Klose, Camerer, Somerfeld, Steinitz, Ohlmuller and others which form the basis of the revision made by Garrow [14]. From these authors, it can be concluded that although the undernourished has lost a lot of weight, even more is lost in solid than in water, and that these patients have, in relative values, more water than the newborns.

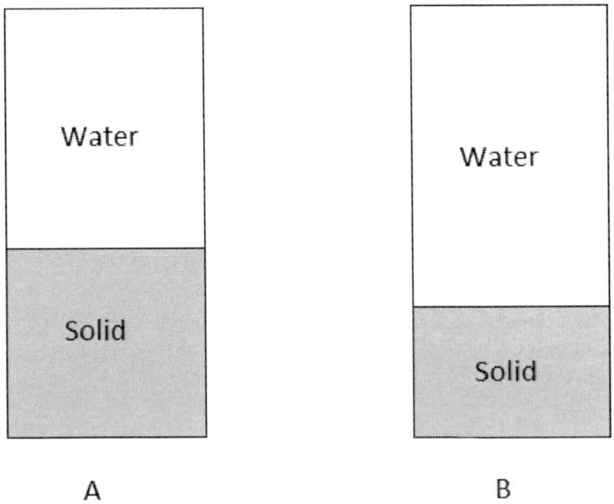

Figure 2. The relative composition of the body of the eutrophic and malnourished child. A. Eutrophic child. B. Malnourished child.

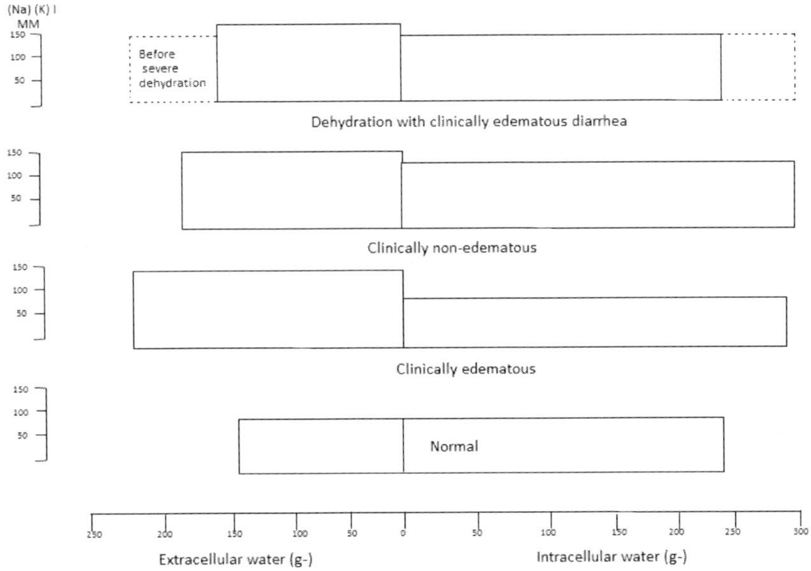

Figure 3. Muscle composition in advanced malnutrition. (Data per 100 g of fat-free solids). The ordinates indicate concentrations of sodium in the extracellular fluid and potassium in the intracellular. In the upper diagram the dotted lines express the composition of the muscle observed before an episode of severe electrolytic imbalance occurred, and the continuous ones, corresponding to the course of the latter.

Better studies by German pediatricians in the field of chemical anatomy of the malnourished have eliminated any doubt about the existence of "dilution" in this disease [15]. From these data, it can be concluded that water represents 78% of the "weight free of water" in the normal child, while in the third-grade malnourished, the figures vary between 81 and 87%. (Figure 3).

Thus, it can be said that dilution and atrophy are indeed "anatomical" expressions of the pathology of the malnourished and that life in that somatic reality is only possible by complicated homeostatic adjustments of the patient's physiology.

Blood Proteins

If it is considered that in the metabolic exchange of tissues, circulating albumins indirectly translate the protein content of the tissues, then, the concentration of a protein in the plasma will depend on the balance between synthesis, distribution in the organism and loss either by catabolism or elimination [12].

The albumin is schematically equal in and out of the vascular space and for its concentration in the plasma to remain constant, it must also be constant in the extravascular space. However, of the biochemical alterations observed in malnutrition, hypoalbuminemia is the most characteristic. In this case, it is due to deficient synthesis that originates from the deficient, incomplete and unbalanced supply of amino acids, through a diet that most of the time is exclusively vegetable. Since deficient synthesis leads to the depletion of tissue proteins, this will result in an alteration in plasma levels.

Albumin

Total body albumin is reduced by 50% in Kwashiorkor patients, with the reduction being proportionally larger in extravascular space. These phenomena seem to be contingent on the intensity and chronicity of the negative nitrogen balance and also relate to dilution. They may also be highly responsible for the onset of edema when we considered that in the pathophysiology of this sign blood proteins are only one of the conditioning factors. The basic differences in the seroprotein pattern of third-grade malnourished with or without edema lie in the levels of albumin and alpha globulins. Therefore, the existence or absence of edema has to relate to them, rather than to other protein fractions [16].

Total Proteins

In third-grade malnourished, total blood serum proteins were found to be below normal levels and less than in non-edematous infants and older edematous children. The information thus gathered, evidently demonstrates a new biochemical and functional balance in the malnourished. The gradual elevation of gamma-globulins, the presence of the same level of beta-globulins, the decrease of albumins, and the different behavior of alpha-globulins in the edematous and non-edematous children firmly established that in the third-grade malnourished, there is no moment - neither because of their age nor because of the chronicity of the ailment - in which the pattern of blood proteins is equal to or corresponding to the normal pattern of a given age and so, should be considered as a resultant or expression of detention of growth and development.

Enzymatic Changes

Different alterations of the enzymatic systems in the liver vary in their response to malnutrition in experimental models with animals. The enzymes in the urea cycle are enhanced by a high protein diet. Leucine-degrading enzymes decreased in rats fed with low-protein diets.

Rats feeding with a low protein diet caused a drop in cytochrome P-450 and when phenobarbital was administered, the cytochrome P-450 level increased only to 25% of the level found in rats treated with Phenobarbital, but with an adequate diet [17].

Da Silva Faria started a research on drug metabolism in young rats chronically fed with low-protein diets, which simulated the value of dietary proteins used by children in areas where caloric-protein malnutrition was prevalent [18]. The results showed that the livers of chronically malnourished rats have a decreased capacity of the oxidative microsomes that metabolize the drugs. By adding hexobarbital, the hepatic microsomes of the malnourished animals showed a less intense spectral change than the microsomes of the age-matched controls that were well fed. The cytochrome P-450 concentration was reduced while the activities of the reductase enzymes - cytochrome b5 concentration, NADPH-cytochrome c reductase and NADPH-cytochrome P-450, were maintained. Administration of phenobarbital, a known enzyme inducer, increased cytochrome P-450, NADPH-cytochrome c reductase activity, NADPH-cytochrome p-450 reductase activity, and increased the magnitude of spectral change.

The descriptions suggest that there is a reduction in the binding of the substrate to the cytochrome P-450 which precedes the oxidative enzymatic reaction, explained by the reduction of the metabolism of the drug in vitro in microsomes of rats fed with low protein diet.

PHARMACOKINETIC CHANGES IN MALNOURISHED CHILDREN

Malnutrition is often a complex process in which many deficiencies occur simultaneously. The changes occur in almost every organ in the body. Apart from the pathophysiological changes that occur with caloric-protein malnutrition, the deficiencies of vitamins, minerals and trace elements are accompanied by various metabolic changes in the tissues.

As a consequence, there is a great potential to alter drug response in malnutrition, not only in the possible changes in drug kinetics, but also in the changes that occur in the entry and location of drugs in the tissues as well as potential alteration in drug-receptor interactions.

There are very few studies on the kinetics and pharmacodynamics of drugs in malnutrition states in human populations [19], thus it is obligatory to study the systematic evaluation of both pharmacokinetics and pharmacodynamics, especially with drugs having a wide range of different physicochemical and pharmacokinetic properties. This multi-deficiency syndrome can alter pharmacokinetic processes as a consequence of disorders in the digestive system, renal function, distribution of liquids in different body compartments, as well as enzymatic disorders at the liver level, some of which have to do with biotransformation. Also important are the deficiencies of some vitamins whose role is important in the activation of such systems. Hence, it is not surprising that severe caloric-protein malnutrition may alter pharmacokinetic processes, as well as pharmacological response and drug toxicity.

Disease States That Alter Pharmacokinetics

The diseases and their severity can dramatically influence the establishment of optimal treatment regimens. It was also established that there are greater knowledge that would help to understand how these factors can influence drug therapy as well as to understand some origins of pharmacokinetic variation and pharmacodynamics.

By definition, diseases are processes that alter the normal functions of the organism. These alterations lead to the manifestations of the disease because the body handles much more drugs and endogenous substances as well as the pharmacokinetics of drugs in common use in the same way. For example, renal failure produces an accumulation of endogenous substances as drugs that are normally excreted by this route. Similarly, diseases that impair the ability of the liver to metabolize and excrete endogenous substances may also have the same effect on drugs, although this process in the liver is more difficult to define when compared with the case of the kidney. Heart failure and other pathological conditions compromising cardiac function can reduce blood perfusion of tissues where absorption, metabolism, distribution and excretion are performed and can profoundly alter the timing and arrangement of many drugs. Also changes in drug binding to proteins could change the availability of drugs as well as drug-receptor interaction [20].

JUSTIFICATION AND IMPORTANCE OF PHARMACOKINETIC STUDIES IN MALNOURISHED CHILDREN

It is well known that the therapeutic response to a drug depends on a variety of factors such as absorption, tissue distribution, tissue response and rate of drug clearance. Elimination processes depend on factors such as biotransformation processes, plasma binding and/or tissue proteins and renal clearance. There are some reports in the literature that point out the effects of malnutrition on these factors, particularly on the liver enzymes, drug metabolizers [19], however, the largest information comes from studies in experimental animals.

Because the cytochrome P-450 hepatic enzyme system is of considerable importance in determining the effect of drugs, pesticides, and chemical carcinogens on animals, any alteration in the system produced by low-protein diets may be of importance in humans, especially those living on low protein diets. The observations that oxidative drug metabolism is markedly reduced in young rats fed with low-protein diets similar to diets consumed by children where caloric-protein malnutrition is prevalent suggest that, in an important form, humans could metabolize foreign compounds at a reduced rate.

The above made us to look for models that would enable us to study enzymatic systems in vivo and hence the possibility to study the enzymatic functionality in humans. For this purpose, the reactions of phase I (oxidation) were explored using the pharmacokinetics of antipyrine and the pharmacokinetics of metronidazole, which is regulated by the functionality of two different isoenzymes belonging to the cytochrome P-450; and the reactions of phase II (conjugation) with the pharmacokinetics of chloramphenicol which is regulated by the enzymatic activity of glucuronyl transferase. To explore renal excretion in patients with severe malnutrition, we made recourse to the pharmacokinetic studies of drugs that are eliminated exclusively by the kidney and which do not undergo biotransformation, as is the case of aminoglycosides.

Because organic alterations caused by severe malnutrition; among which the changes in the biochemical composition as well as the disorders in those apparatus and systems that have to do with the kinetic processes of absorption, distribution, biotransformation and excretion both of the original drug and of its metabolites and/or xenobiotic agents; suggest that the malnourished child is a subject with a high risk of intoxication or of therapeutic ineffectiveness if they are managed with the same treatment schemes used in children without malnutrition.

The above made it necessary to conduct studies on the metabolism of drugs in patients suffering from severe malnutrition. Although there are research oriented reports in the literature to know these aspects, it should be pointed out that the largest pairs have been performed in adults and very few in patients of pediatric age, although this population turns out to be the most affected.

Based on the above, it was considered pertinent to carry out this line of research, which aimed to obtain more information about the effects of severe malnutrition on some pathways of elimination such as: some metabolic pathways and renal excretion of some drugs of common use.

Clinical Utility of Pharmacokinetic Studies

The knowledge obtained from the pharmacokinetic studies would confirm whether alterations of drug metabolizing enzymes due to undernutrition, demonstrated both in vitro and in experimental models in animals, are also altered in humans. Likewise, with these studies, it will be possible to predict from pharmacokinetic knowledge, and using simulation models, the repercussion of chronic exposure to a commonly used drug that requires the same routes of elimination.

On the other hand, knowledge of the functionality of the metabolic pathways for biotransformation and drug elimination through pharmacokinetic studies leads to a more rational use of drugs in pediatric populations where the prevalence of malnutrition continues to be high. The pharmacokinetic results obtained could be used for the purpose of optimizing therapeutic regimens by individualizing the dose and increasing the pharmacokinetic studies with other therapeutic drugs, in order to improve the efficacy and safety of the drugs. Intra- and inter-individual variability in the pharmacokinetics of most drugs is determined, in an important way, by liver function variables, as has already been described by blood flow parameters to the liver and metabolic capacity. These parameters may be altered as a result of diseases affecting the liver, genetic differences in drug metabolizing enzymes and various types of drug interactions, including the involvement of induction and inhibition enzymes or low regularization.

With the now known large number of drug metabolizing enzymes, their differential substrate specificity and their differential induction or inhibition capacity for each test substance to measure liver function, should be used as a functional test to identify their specific metabolizing enzyme. Thus the concept of the test substance model provides general information about the severe limitations that the usual liver function tests have. To test the metabolic activity of various enzymes, test substances can be given or various metabolites of a single test substance can also be analyzed. The analysis of enzyme-specific as a test of liver function is more preferable to the analysis of metabolites than analysis of the clearance test of the unchanged substance. At least 5 different types of cytochrome P-450 induction enzymes may be within the variability of liver function. This may be quantified by biochemical parameters, purification methods or highly specific methods such as Western blot analysis, which comprises molecular biology techniques such as quantification of mRNA in blood and tissues.

Therapeutic drug monitoring is implicitly used for the quantification of enzyme activities relevant to a specific drug, when the maximum and minimum plasma concentration in the steady state is available. Selective damage of liver enzymes, as determined by gene mutations, may have an effect on the pharmacokinetics of certain drugs, similar to that caused by liver cirrhosis. The evaluation of this variability of hereditary origin in hepatic cirrhosis is possible thanks to *in vivo* and *ex vivo* enzymatic methods.

For genetically polymorphic enzymes and the carrier proteins involved in drug delivery, molecular genetic methods that use patient blood samples can be used to classify individuals into: (i) impaired or poor metabolizers (homozygous deficient); (ii) the group of large metabolizers (deficient homozygotes) and (iii) the group of extensive metabolizers (heterozygotes).

The evaluation of liver function primarily denotes the consideration of biochemical parameters, such as the parameters of liver cell destruction (aminotransferases) and synthetic liver functions (coagulation parameters, serum albumin) and metabolic parameters (bilirubin) [21, 22]. These parameters and the chemical evaluation of the patient can provide a routine estimation of liver function. This can be expressed operationally by the patient classification score [23].

Secondly, compounds of test models are applicable and provide quantitative information on liver metabolic function [24]. The metabolism of these test substances should not be subject to genetic polymorphism [25]. These were also classified as providers of information regarding hepatic blood flow when their liver extraction rate was above 0.7 or dependent on liver metabolic capacity if their liver extraction rate was less than 0.3. The test substances can also be classified as indicators of either phase I or phase II metabolism. It should be borne in mind that the specificity of the enzymes of hepatic metabolism implies that no substance of the general model can be predictive for most drugs.

This finding is increasing considerably in the practice of liver function tests because by the use of isolated enzymes and genetically modified cell lines, enzymes relevant to certain drugs can now be specifically analyzed [26]. Recent knowledge makes it possible to understand the role of the specific enzyme in drug-drug interactions including inhibition, down-regulation or induction of enzymes and prediction of clinically relevant genetic polymorphisms.

Technically, both the depuration methods (pharmacokinetic profile) as well as the proportions between drug concentrations and their metabolites in blood and urine are calculated as indicators of certain metabolic activities. The *in vivo* tests for specific enzymes that differ predominantly for genetic reasons, is called phenotyping. The methods of genotyping make the prognosis of the enzyme activity in the metabolism of drugs possible and provide a basis for molecular genetics.

Cytochrome P-450 Enzymes and the Mixed-Function Oxygenase System

Many drugs and other chemicals are metabolized in the liver primarily by the hepatic mixed-function oxidase system before they are excreted from the body. The mixed-function oxidase system receives electrons from NADPH or NADH. Reduced equivalents are then transferred through cytochrome P450-NADPH reductase to cytochrome p450 hemoproteins. Cytochrome b5 is a component of the system in the metabolism of some substrates. The formation of a cytochrome P450 complex, an oxygen-molecule, and a chemical substrate precedes the transfer of one oxygen atom to the substrate to form the product and the other atom to form H_2O. Many P450 proteins, cDNAs, and genes have been isolated and sequenced. The term P450 collectively refers to a superfamily of individual P450 enzymes. P450 forms, found primarily in the liver, have been classified into 4 gene families, designated I to IV, based primarily on their amino acid sequence. The subfamilies are designated by the sequence of capital letters and genes within a family by Arabic numerals. P450 enzymes are conjugated by other enzymes in the cytosol and endoplasmic reticulum, which form glucuronides, sulfate, glutathione and other conjugates [27]. In general, the enzymes of the P450 complex are possibly more inducible by environmental factors than in the conjugating enzymes.

INTER-SPECIES DIFFERENCES AND EFFECTS OF DIET ON CYTOCHROME P450 ENZYMES

Many studies about the effects of dietary composition and nutritional deficiencies in the metabolism of drugs and other chemical substances in animals were carried out earlier for several P450 isoforms that had been identified and characterized. The interpretation of some studies may have been complicated by extreme dietary variations leading to other pathological processes [28].

Procedures such as overnight fasting before killing animals, or feeding in pairs that may involve prolonged periods of fasting to control animals, may also complicate the interpretation. It is difficult to extrapolate results from studies of mixed-function oxidases system performed in animals to humans. The differences between species of P450 enzymes in the rates of drug metabolism and in toxicity and resistance to various chemicals may be substantial. Studies to identify dietary components that may influence drug metabolism in humans have been conducted mostly in healthy individuals who consumed nutritionally adequate diets under controlled conditions.

This approach is more likely to provide clear and consistent information on the effect of specific dietary changes that have been studied in patients in whom delineated diseases, concurrent therapy and many other factors possibly influence outcomes. However, although the studies which have been conducted in patient populations are few, they have suggested that changes in diet and nutritional status have important influences on drug metabolism.

Other Food Effects on Drug Metabolism

The effects of diet and nutritional status on the post-absorptive metabolism of drugs and other chemicals by enzymes of the P450 complex are extremely important. Foods may also influence gastrointestinal absorption and bioavailability of chemicals [29]. Bioavailability may be altered by the direct binding of a drug to certain substances contained in foods or by altering luminal pH, gastric emptying, intestinal transit, absorption through the gastrointestinal mucosa and Hepatosplenic blood flow.

In part, foods may induce changes in the bioavailability of some drugs by altering the mechanisms of liver clearance or by competing with drugs for first-step metabolism in the intestine. Drugs can undergo metabolic transformation by microorganisms in the intestine [30]. Consequently, the influence of diet on the gastrointestinal flora may alter the intestinal metabolism of some drugs.

Effects of Macronutrients of Diet, Fasting and Energy Restriction

Protein Diet

Significant evidence indicates that dietary protein may influence the cytochrome P450 enzyme complex. For instance, in male and female rats fed with diets for 2 weeks in which the protein content varied from 5 to 50%, there was an increase in the toxicity of pentobarbital and strychnine and a reduction of the *in vivo* metabolism of barbiturates by protein [31].

The metabolism of pentobarbital, strychnine, aminopyrin, oxazolamine and aniline by hepatic microsomes, went down by a lower protein intake. The effects were more marked for the first 3 substances. Most of the effects of dietary restriction on protein were more marked in the male animals.

Flavoprotein reductase and cytochrome b5 decreased somewhat by protein restriction. No clear difference was observed by sex. In this study, glucose was isocalorically replaced by casein. The rats with high protein intake gained weight, while those with low protein intake consumed less energy. Nevertheless, this study demonstrated a dose-response relationship between dietary proteins and activities of mixed-function hepatic oxidases.

Inducibility of cytochrome P450 by phenobarbital in rats is also reduced by decreased protein intake. The effects of diets containing primarily poor quality proteins on the enzymes of the P450 enzyme complex are similar to the effects of protein restrictions. Protein deficiency in female monkeys may reduce hepatic P450 levels, but other components of the mixed-function oxidase system and some associated enzymatic activities are less affected in this species than in rats.

The toxic effects of a large number of chemicals that are inactivated by the mixed-function oxidase system in the liver are increased by protein restriction. Among the substances involved are pesticides that include endosulfan, captan, lindane and diazinon when administered to weaned rats with a kwashiorkor-like condition [32].

Effects of Serious Malnutrition on Phase I Reactions

Pharmacokinetics of Antipyrine

The most widely used marker for hepatic oxidation capacity has been antipyrine [33]. This drug is rapidly and almost completely absorbed from the gut and does not have a significant preservative metabolism. It is distributed in body water and has plasma protein bindings of only 10%. 95% is metabolized by liver microsomal mixed-function monooxygenase enzymes and the 3 main products are norgenazone, 3-hydroxymethy-lantipyrine and 4-hydroxyanpyrine. Likewise, 3 different cytochrome P450 enzymes are possibly involved in the metabolism of antipyrine, although the available data allow a vague classification of it as CYPIA2, CYP2C and CYP3A. CYPIA2 may be involved in the formation of 4-hydroxyantipyrine.

The metabolism of antipyrine is a reliable index of hepatic microsomal oxidative function. Its plasma half-life is inversely proportional to the activity of the enzymes. It is metabolized almost entirely in the liver by hydroxylation to 3 metabolites which are finally excreted in the urine. Only a fraction of the drug from the plasma follows first-order kinetics. The nontoxic nature and its metabolic characteristics make its pharmacokinetic study an excellent model for evaluating the hepatic microsomal system.

In one of the first studies on the pharmacokinetics of antipyrine in malnourished children [34], found that the elimination half-life was longer in children with severe malnutrition, which was determined by decreased total clearance. With nutritional rehabilitation for 4 to 9 weeks, both changes can be reversed, indicating that the adverse effects of severe caloric-protein malnutrition (SCPM) on liver microsomal oxidation are reversible. Also observed an increase in elimination half-life and a decrease in the clearance rate in 8 non-edematous children with severe malnutrition. Re-evaluation after 3 to 4 weeks of good nutrition showed an impressive decrease in half-life and an increase in the rate of clearance.

In addition to the decreased half-life of antipyrine clearance and clearance rate in patients with kwashiorkor malnutrition, they demonstrated an improvement in the excretion of D-glutaric acid which is an indirect index of liver microsomal activity. They also documented that excretion of the metabolites of antipyretic; 4-hydroxyanpyridine, norantipyrine, 3-hydroxymethylantipyrine and carboxyantipirine; were increased in 5 children with kwashiorkor after having been properly fed for 3 weeks.

The finding in our study, consisted in the identification of lower clearance rates in the malnourished than in the same children during their rehabilitation, which speaks in favor of alterations in the mechanisms that modulate the elimination of the drug as an explanation of the extension of the elimination half-life [34].

The use of TCOM in a similar study, performed by the group in 6 children with SCPM, permits the addition of two more facts to the studies of antipyrine pharmacokinetics in malnourished patients. The first is a decrease in the volume of distribution in steady state (Vdss) and with the transfer rate constant from the central compartment to the periphery, K12 decreased during the stage of severe malnutrition. The second is the concomitant increase in the transfer rate constant from the peripheral compartment to the central unit K21 during nutritional recovery. The explanation of these findings could be owed to the decrease of effective concentrations of the drug in the extravascular and intravascular spaces, which in the case of other medicines as some antibiotics to which pharmacokinetics were similar, could have therapeutic meaning.

From a dosing regimen point of view, the results show that it is not sufficient to know the concentrations of a drug in blood or plasma and its rate of elimination, but also it is necessary to obtain the blood re-exchange transference micro-constants o the compartments where it is required to act.

With the objective of establishing the possible relationship of each of the pharmacokinetic values with the biological variables such as age, weight and height, linear regression analysis was performed without finding a significant association. The percentage ratio of weight to height as an indicator of nutritional risk did not show any significant correlation with any of the pharmacokinetic parameters of antipyrine. It is therefore proposed as an explanation, that the deficient elimination of drugs is due to the alterations found during malnutrition, which were not totally corrected in the rehabilitation.

Pharmacokinetics of Metronidazole

Metronidazole is an antimicrobial drug, which has been postulated as a test for the study of cytochrome P450 activity. Previous studies in humans and in rats suggest that different cytochromes P450 metabolize metronidazole and also the already established test drug "the antipyrine."

Thus, to know the capacity of drug metabolism, the simultaneous use of these 2 drugs in a cocktail for non-invasive studies have been suggested [35].

Metronidazole is hydroxylated in the microsomes of human livers by a NADPH-dependent process, and possibly catalyzed by the cytochrome P450 system most of the time. Pretreatment of rat hepatocytes with 3-methylcholanthrene increased the speed and affinity of metronidazole hydroxylation and its inhibition by a naphthoflavone. This suggests that cytochrome P450 1A1 and/or 1A2 has a high affinity for hydroxylation of metronidazole [36]. In a recent description using the polymorphism of long restriction fragments, it is pointed out that CYP 1A1 codes for the cytochrome P450 enzyme, an aryl hydrocarbon hydroxylase.

The pharmacokinetics of metronidazole varies in terms of chronological age, as shown by the differences between neonates, and older children, and in young adults and the elderly. It also varies in different disease states, according to their severity. Thus, in patients with severe hepatic disease, systemic clearance of metronidazole was reduced by 66% compared to healthy controls. The severity of the disease status in septicemic children also showed alterations in the pharmacokinetics of metronidazole [37].

The high frequency of intestinal parasitosis in malnourished children has increased the use of metronidazole. However, there is a lack of knowledge about pharmacokinetics in malnourished children, hence the importance of the pharmacokinetic study of metronidazole in this type of patients.

The main descriptions of the studies carried out showed a significant variation in all the pharmacokinetic parameters among the subjects. This variation can be explained by genetic differences or by biological factors not yet identified. Despite high interindividual variability in both malnourished and rehabilitated children, data show that the elimination half-life (t1/2el) increases in severely malnourished children compared to the values obtained in rehabilitated subjects. The increase in the elimination half-life is characterized by a concomitant decrease in the clearance. By virtue of these observations, it is acceptable to infer that the enzymatic system responsible for metabolizing metronidazole is not operating at an optimal rate in children undergoing SCPM. In summary, the pharmacokinetics of metronidazole in severely malnourished children is significantly different from that found in rehabilitated subjects with SCPM as well as in pediatric patients who were not malnourished.

EFFECT OF SEVERE MALNUTRITION ON PHASE II REACTIONS

Pharmacokinetics of Chloramphenicol

Chloramphenicol is an antibiotic commonly used in underdeveloped countries. It is frequently used in typhoid fever, bacillary dysentery, meningitis caused by *Haemophilus* and septicemia. It is a highly liposoluble drug and rapidly absorbed in the gastrointestinal tract, and is well distributed in the body and cerebrospinal fluids [38]. Its body clearance is related to the biotransformation to water soluble glucuronides. This process is carried out by hepatocytes with the assistance of specific enzymes such as glucuronyl transferase enzyme. The metabolites are excreted by the kidneys.

The frequent use of this drug in severe infections where malnutrition is prevalent has been recognized and has hastened its study in patients suffering from malnutrition [39].

In children with SCPM, the drug could be detected in serum for up to 30 hours after dosing compared to 8-12 hours in controls. As a consequence, the area under the ABC curve increased, reflecting increased exposure to chloramphenicol. In normal children, the peak values for chloramphenicol were achieved at 2 hours and reached a minimum concentration at 12 hours. The proportion of its conjugated to unconjugated formation was lower in the urine of malnourished children. Liver biopsies were performed in 2 patients analyzing the activity of bilirubin-UDP glucoronyl transferase enzyme with the finding that this activity was lower in children with severe malnutrition than in healthy adults. Protein deficiency was recently reported in weaned newborn rats with increased glucuronidation of p-nitrophenol [40].

The monitoring of chloramphenicol plasma levels at steady-state, corrected for multi-doses, in 365 nutritionally compromised children who received the drug either orally (14 children) or intravenously (12 children) for treatment of infectious diseases showed significant differences in chloramphenicol plasma concentrations at steady-state in children who had mild malnutrition compared to those who had severe malnutrition.

It is noteworthy that in both oral and intravenous administration, the concentrations achieved in patients with SCPM were close to toxic levels. In contrast to the previous results, our observations indicate that there are no statistically significant pharmacokinetic differences. However, children who had been malnourished and who had recovered from SCPM showed slightly higher plasma concentrations with the areas under the curve (AUC), without reaching statistically significant differences.

The t1/2 and Kel were similar in both severe malnutrition stage and during nutritional recovery. Therefore, our observations indicate that in Mexican children with SCPM, the activity of the enzyme chloramphenicol-UDP glucoronyl tranferase is not significantly altered in patients with severe malnutrition.

Effect of Serious Malnutrition on the Renal Excretion of Drugs

Pharmacokinetics of Gentamicin

Gentamicin sulfate is a bactericidal antibiotic of the group of aminoglycosides derived from *Microspora Purpurea*. It is active against a number of gram-positive and gram-negative bacteria. Clinically, it is used primarily against *Pseudomonas*, *Proteus* and *Klebsiella Enterobacter* group.

The introduction of gentamicin in medical practice has contributed significantly to the fight against severe infections. The principal route, if not the exclusive way, for its elimination of gentamicin is the kidneys through glomerular filtration [41]. However, from previous studies, it is known that on the first day of therapy, 40% of the administered dose is excreted in the urine, while subsequent days 85% or more are excreted, suggesting an initial accumulation or dilution of equilibrium within the body that is relatively independent of renal function. Other studies also indicated that approximately 30% of gentamicin in plasma is protein bound.

Gentamicin is not absorbed when given orally, however it is readily absorbed when administered intramuscularly. It is eliminated in the same way as penicillins, except its binding to proteins is insignificant [42].

Its elimination half-life was longer in children with kwashiorkor during admission to the hospital (229.0 ± 94.8 minutes) than during their nutritional recovery. The purification increased from 13.6 ± 6.0 mL/min to 28.7 ± 21.3 mL/min. These alterations were accompanied by a decrease in the half-life of the paraminohipurate, and an increase in the apparent volume of distribution, which spans from 3.9 ± 0.46 L to 5.53 ± 11.0 L. On the other hand, the pharmacokinetics of intravenous gentamicin in children with marasmus did not reveal any difference in the distribution and/or elimination of the drug. The implications of these observations on therapeutic efficacy or on toxicity such as nephrotic or ototoxicity require additional studies with multiple doses. At present, it is not possible to establish definitive recommendations for dose or dose intervals for children with SCPM. However, another important variable is the binding of the drug to plasma proteins. Three widely used antibiotics showed significant changes in their binding to plasma proteins therefore, more than 10 to 15% of the drug is available in free form. On the other hand, both penicillin and gentamicin showed no similarities in the two stages of the study, which discards the possibility of damage to the renal elimination pathway due to severe malnutrition. Although heart failure is relatively rare, there is evidence that the cardiovascular system is affected in severe malnutrition [43]. Bradycardia, low blood pressure and cyanosis have been reported, the heart is small and there are signs of circulatory insufficiency. These changes may be indirectly responsible for decreased renal plasma flow, with a consequent reduction in glomerular filtration. These functional changes make us to suspect alterations in the pharmacokinetics of drugs excreted by the renal route. However, in the results obtained by us on the pharmacokinetics of gentamicin, despite the reduction in blood flow to the kidney and glomerular filtration, it appears that they are not sufficiently altered by the effects of severe malnutrition to modify the pharmacokinetics of drugs that are excreted by glomerular filtration. In order to ensure the absence of pharmacokinetic differences that could be observed with compartmental models, we performed the analysis with non-compartmental models with the finding that the mentioned observations persisted, which strengthens the results obtained.

CONCLUSION

1) SCPM alters the oxidative pathway corresponding to Phase I reactions by reducing the capacity of the participating enzyme systems. Decreased metabolic clearance and prolongation of the half-life of antipyrine clearance in children with SCPM indicate a decrease in the functional capacity of the CYPIA2, CYP2C and CYP3A enzyme systems responsible for antipyrine bio-transformation. Decreased metabolic clearance and prolongation of the mean elimination half-life of metronidazole in children with SCPM indicate a decrease in the functional capacity of the CYP1A1 and/or CYPIA2 enzyme systems responsible for the biotransformation of metronidazole.
2) Hepatic conjugation mechanisms dependent on Phase II reactions, in which the enzyme glucuronyl transferase participates, are not altered by the effect of SCPM, since the pharmacokinetics of chloramphenicol were not different in the same patients during severe nutrition and during their nutritional recovery.

3) Renal excretion of drugs in which glomerular filtration mechanisms are involved is not altered by the effect of SCPM, since the pharmacokinetics of gentamicin was not different in children with SCPM in the acute stage and during their nutritional recovery.
4) The previous results were confirmed, using compartmental and non-compartmental models.
5) The reduction of the oxidative capacity in the biotransformation of drugs in patients with SCPM requires reducing the dose and/or extending the intervals of administration of those drugs that are eliminated by this route, in order to improve their efficacy and safety.
6) Because of the interindividual variability in the pharmacokinetics of the studied drugs, it is advisable to individualize the therapeutic regimens, if we want to optimize its therapeutic management in pediatric patients who are under severe malnutrition.

REFERENCES

[1] Shamah-Levy T, Mundo-Rosas V, Morales-Ruan C, Cuevas-Nasu L, Méndez-Gómez-Humarán I, Pérez-Escamilla R. Food insecurity and maternal-child nutritional status in Mexico: cross-sectional analysis of the National Health and Nutrition Survey 2012. *BMJ.* Open. 2017;7:e014371

[2] Vallejo KP, Martínez CM, Matos Adames AA, Fuchs-Tarlovsky V, Nogales GCC, Paz RER, Perman MI, Correia MITD, Waitzberg DL. Current clinical nutrition practices in critically ill patients in Latin America: a multinational observational study. *Crit Care.* 2017;21:227.

[3] Valdez López RM, Fausto Guerra J, Valadez FI, Ramos Ramos A, Loreto Garibay O, Villaseñor Farias M. [Nutritional state and shortcoming of micronutrients on schooled youth's diet on the

metropolitan zone of Guadalajara Jalisco]. *Arch Latinoam Nutr.* 2012;62:161-6.

[4] Bonetti L, Terzoni S, Lusignani M, Negri M, Froldi M, Destrebecq A. Prevalence of malnutrition among older people in medical and surgical wards in hospital and quality of nutritional care: a multicenter, cross-sectional study. *J Clin Nurs*. 2017 Aug 22.

[5] Suri S, Kumar D, Das R. Dietary deficiency of vitamin A among rural children: A community-based survey using a food-frequency questionnaire. *Natl. Med J India.* 2017; 30:61-64.

[6] Lima AA, Leite ÁM, Di Moura A, Lima NL, Soares AM, Abreu CB, Filho JQ, Mota RM, Lima IF, Havt A, Medeiros PH, Prata MM, Guedes MM, Cavalcante PA, Veras HN, Santos AK, Moore SR, Pinkerton RC, Houpt ER, Guerrant RL. Determinant Variables, Enteric Pathogen Burden, Gut Function, and Immune-Related Inflammatory Biomarkers Associated with Childhood Malnutrition: A Prospective Case-Control Study in North eastern Brazil. *Pediatr Infect Dis J.* 2017 Feb 22.

[7] Yakoob MY, Lo CW. Nutrition (Micronutrients) in Child Growth and Development: A Systematic Review on Current Evidence, Recommendations and Opportunities for Further Research. *J Dev Behav Pediatr.* 2017 Jul 25.

[8] Müller MJ, Enderle J, Pourhassan M, Braun W, Eggeling B, Lagerpusch M, Glüer CC, Kehayias JJ, Kiosz D, Bosy-Westphal A. Metabolic adaptation to caloric restriction and subsequent refeeding: the Minnesota Starvation Experiment revisited. *Am J Clin. Nutr.* 2015;102:807-19.

[9] Ramos GR. *Homeorrhesis as a phenomenon of adaptation to calorie protein deficiency.* Protein Advisory Group. WHO/FAOINICEF. Ginebra 1966.

[10] Jorde R, Sneve M, Figenschau Y, Svartberg J, Waterloo K. Effects of vitamin D supplementation on symptoms of depression in overweight and obese subjects: randomized double blind trial. *J Intern Med.* 2008;264:599-609.

[11] Jolliffe DA, Griffiths CJ, Martineau AR. Vitamin D in the prevention of acute respiratory infection: systematic review of clinical studies. *J Steroid Biochem Mol Biol.* 2013;136:321-9.

[12] Zhu K, Oddy WH, Holt P, Ping-Delfos WCS, Mountain J, Lye S, Pennell C, Hart PH, Walsh JP. Tracking of vitamin D status from childhood to early adulthood and its association with peak bone mass. *Am J Clin. Nutr.* 2017;106:276-283.

[13] Mpio I, Cleaud C, Arkouche W, Laville M. [Results of therapeutics strategy of protein-energy wasting in chronic hemodialysis: a prospective study during 12 months]. *Nephrol. Ther.* 2015;11:97-103.

[14] Garrow JS, Smith R, Ward EE. *Electrolyte metabolism in severe infantile malnutrition*. Oxford: Pergamon Press, 1968.

[15] Bandsma RH, Mendel M, Spoelstra MN, Reijngoud DJ, Boer T, Stellaard F, Brabin B, Schellekens R, Senga E, Heikens GT. Mechanisms behind decreased endogenous glucose production in malnourished children. *Pediatr Res.* 2010;68:423-8.

[16] Lee JL, Oh ES, Lee RW, Finucane TE. Serum Albumin and Prealbumin in Calorically Restricted, Non diseased Individuals: A Systematic Review. *Am J Med.* 2015;128:1023.

[17] Jung D, Prasad PP. Influence of nutritional status on the pharmacokinetics and pharmacodynamics of pentobarbital. *Drug Metab Dispos.* 1989;17:365-8.

[18] da Silva Faria T, da Fonte Ramos C, Sampaio FJ. Puberty onset in the female offspring of rats submitted to protein or energy restricted diet during lactation. *J Nutr Biochem.* 2004;15:123-7.

[19] Earl-Salotti GI, Charland SL. The effect of parenteral nutrition on hepatic cytochrome P-450. *JPEN J Parenter Enteral Nutr.* 1994; 18:458-65.

[20] Abe Y, Ota E, Endo T, Murakami M, Kobayashi M. Absorption, disposition, metabolism, and excretion of ritobegron (KUC-7483), a novel selective β3-adrenoceptor agonist, in rats. *Pharmazie.* 2014; 69:881-8.

[21] Goldberg DM, Brown D. Advances in the application of biochemical test to disease of the liver and biliary tract: their role in diagnosis and the elucidation of pathogenic mechanism. *Clin Biochem* 1987; 20:127.

[22] Johnson PJ. Role of the standard "Liver function test" in the current clinical practice. *Ann Clin Biochem* 1989; 26:463.

[23] Howden CW, Birnic GG, Brodie MJ. Drug metabolism in liver disease. *Pharmacol. Ther* 1989; 40:439.

[24] Vesell ES. *The model drug approach in clinical pharmacology*. 1991; 50:239.

[25] Wilkinson GR. Clearance approaches in pharmacology. *Pharmacol Rev* 1987; 39:1.

[26] Fuht U, Dochmer J, Battula N. Biotransformation of caffeine and theophylline in mammalian cells lines genetically engineered for expression of single cytochrome p450 isoforms. *Biochem Pharmacol* 1992; 43:225.

[27] Yang CS, Yoo JSH. Dietary effects on drug metabolism by the mixed function oxidase system. *Pharmacol. Ther* 1988; 38:253.

[28] Ning M, Jeong H. High-Fat Diet Feeding Alters Expression of Hepatic Drug-Metabolizing Enzymes in Mice. *Drug Metab Dispos.* 2017;45:707-711.

[29] Roe DA. Diet nutrition and drug reactions. In Shils NF, Young VR. *8thed Modern Nutrition in Health and Disease*. Lea & Febiger. Philadelphia: 1994, p 630-45.

[30] Liedholm H, Melander A. Concomitant food intake can increase the bioavailability of propranolol by transient inhibition of its presystemic primary conjugation. *Clin Pharmacol Ther* 1986; 40:29.

[31] Segawa R, Hayashi H, Morita R, Ogawa T, Takimoto N, Hara S, Suzuki K, Shibutani M, Mitsumori K. Modifying effects of liver tumor promotion in rats subjected toco-administration of indole-3-carbinol and phenobarbital. *J Toxicol Sci.* 2014;39:129-40.

[32] Benjamin N, Kushwah A, Sharma RK, Katiyar AK. Histo-pathological changes in liver, kidney and muscles of pesticides

exposed malnourished and diabetic rats. *Indian J Exp Biol.* 2006; 44:228-32.

[33] Sharer JE, Wrighton SA. Identification of the human hepatic cytochromes P450 involved in the in vitro oxidation of antipyrine. *Drug Metab Dispos.* 1996;24:487-94.

[34] Lares-Asseff I, Santiago-Porras MP, Pérez-Ortiz B, Cravioto J. Pharmacokinetics of antipyrine in grade III malnourished children during the acute phase and recovery. *Bol Med Hosp Infant Mex.* 1988;45:298-306.

[35] Loft S. Metronidazole and antipyrine as probes for the study of foreign compounds metabolism. *Pharmacol Toxicol* 1990; 66:1.

[36] Pearce RE, Cohen-Wolkowiez M, Sampson MR, Kearns GL.The role of human cytochrome P450enzymes in the formation of 2-hydroxymetronidazole: CYP2A6 is the high affinity (low Km) catalyst. *Drug Metab Dispos.* 2013; 41:1686-94.

[37] Butler DR, Kuhn RJ, Chandler MH. Pharmacokinetics of anti-infective agents in paediatric patients. *Clin Pharmacokinet.* 1994; 26:374-95.

[38] Sullins AK, Abdel-Rahman SM. Pharmacokinetics of antibacterial agents in the CSF of children and adolescents. *Paediatr Drugs*. 2013; 15:93-117.

[39] Lazzerini M, Tickell D. Antibiotics in severely malnourished children: systematic review of efficacy, safety and pharmacokinetics. *Bull World Health Organ.* 2011; 89:594-607.

[40] Chen M, Howe D, Leduc B, Kerr S, Williams DA. Identification and characterization of two chloramphenicol glucuronides from the in vitro glucuronidation of chloramphenicol in human liver microsomes. *Xenobiotica* 2007; 37:954-71.

[41] De Cock RF, Allegaert K, Brussee JM, Sherwin CM, Mulla H, de Hoog M, van den Anker JN, Danhof M, Knibbe CA. Simultaneous pharmacokinetic modeling of gentamicin, tobramycin and vancomycin clearance from neonates to adults: towards a semi physiological function for maturation in glomerular filtration. *Pharm Res* 2014; 31:2643-54.

[42] Abo El Sooud K. Comparative disposition kinetics and plasma protein binding of gentamic in sulphate in three juvenile animal species. *J Vet Med A Physiol Pathol Clin Med.* 2003; 50:196-200.

[43] Tennant IA, Barnett AT, Thompson DS, Kips J, Boyne MS, Chung EE, Chung AP, Osmond C, Hanson MA, Gluckman PD, Segers P, Cruickshank JK, Forrester TE. Impaired cardiovascular structure and function in adult survivors of severe acute malnutrition. *Hypertension* 2014; 64:664-71.

In: The Optimization of Drug Prescribing … ISBN: 978-1-53612-263-3
Editor: Hugo Juarez Olguin

Chapter 9

PHARMACOVIGILANCE AND PHARMACOEPIDEMIOLOGY OF DRUGS IN A PEDIATRIC HOSPITAL

Hugo Juarez Olguín[1,2,*], Fernanda Reyes Gonzalez[1] and Janett Flores Perez[1,2]
[1]Laboratorio de Farmacología, InstitutoNacional de Pediatría, Mexico City, Mexico
[2]Departamento de Farmacología, Facultad de Medicina, Universidad Nacional Autónoma de México, Mexico City, Mexico

ABSTRACT

Pharmacovigilance (PV) comprises of a series of actions aimed at detecting and registering of Adverse Drug Reactions (ADRs), while pharmacoepidemiology (PE) addresses issues pertaining to all the activities, which involve the detection of drug prescription patterns. We describe the procedures of PV and PE of drugs used in a pediatric

* Corresponding Author Email: juarezol@yahoo.com

hospital. The PV activities show that there is a relation between an increase in the incidence of ADRs and the prescription of a larger number of drugs. The PE activities reveal that antibiotics are the most frequently prescribed drugs followed by drugs used for gastrointestinal diseases. Since PV and PE activities were initiated, they have contributed to an adequate use of drugs in children. When the PE of a hospital is known, drug consumption can be optimally planned. PV and PE demonstrate that when polytherapy is not necessary, it must be avoided. Finally, the present guide can be adopted to initiate PV and PE at any hospital.

INTRODUCTION

The National Institute of Pediatrics of Mexico, a tertiary-care center located in Mexico City, is one of the hospitals of its kind that attends to patients ranging from newborns to teenagers, with diverse health problems in the country. A significant percentage of the patients attended toat the hospital are characterized by presenting chronic and complex diseases of mainly long duration for their late diagnoses, and only a few are patients with recently acquired ailments. In both cases, multiple studies, treatments, hospitalizations, interdisciplinary consultations and long-term follow-up are usually required. Records from the database registry reveal that the Institute provides approximately 200,000 consultations annually with almost 8,000 of this number being hospitalized. The same source shows that more than 6,000 surgical interventions and 500,000 laboratory tests are performed per year in the hospital.

The need for a qualified center that would give specialized support to the activities of pharmacovigilance (PV) and pharmacoepidemiology (PE), regarding the most frequently used pediatric drugs in the hospital, gave birth to the foundation of the Pharmacology Service of the institute and since its creation, the service has thoroughly performed this function. Hence, this chapter aims at describing a procedure for PV and PE for drugs used in a pediatric hospital. Undoubtedly, such activities are very important for their immense contribution in the detection and registration of adverse drug reactions and determination of the patterns of drug prescription in children.

PHARMACOVIGILANCE

The term Adverse Drug Reaction (ADR) describes any harmful and unintentional response to the usual doses of a drug in humans when administered for purposes of prophylaxis, diagnosis, treatment or modification of physiological activities. ADR can be due to hypersensitivity, idiosyncrasy, drug accumulation or pharmacological interactions between two or more drugs.

Most drugs that produce ADR can threaten or worsen the patient's condition. For this reason, PV programs, also called phase IV studies, have been developed to identify ADR, so as to guarantee and ensure drug use safety.

The pharmacology service is a department highly qualified in the detection, notification and registry of ADR caused by medicaments used in hospital [1, 2].

These functions are approached in two dimensions. The first is the collection of patient clinical information and the second is to submit this information to the ADR reference centers of the World Health Organization (WHO).

Certainly, such functions require a multi disciplinary work team within a hospital for efficient detection and registry of ADR which indeed would improve patient attention. An efficient PV program would permit the acquisition of experience and shape the patterns of drug use in the population attended at any health institution, and would enrich the functions of the Hospital Drug Supply Committees in taking effective decisions on drugs to spend their budget, since many hospital centers usually do away with certain types of drugs due to the discovery of resistance and ADR.

Moreover, the constant appearance of new drugs in the market coupled with recent increase in the indiscriminate use of most drugs justifies the necessity of creating a service that would take up the duties of PV. An efficient PV and drug information programs are obvious important sources of knowledge on drugs and necessary tools for a more adequate prescription.

Objectives of the PV Program

PV program objectives should rotate on detection and registration of not only mild but also severe and life-endangering ADRs and their monitoring especially in recently developed drugs. Furthermore, these assignments include the determination of its frequencies, on drug-type bases, in the general population and in particular, in the pediatric population, which is the main target of this work, and establishing the physical-pathological factors predisposing its onset. Moreover, to bring any monitoring work on ADR to completion, the necessity of ADR-data base creation is of paramount importance.

In view of the recent proposals of the Ministry of Health of our country and WHO to develop a national center for the registry of ADRs, the central part of this work is to recollect all these outlined ADR monitoring objectives and put them to work.

Procedure

An effective PE program for ADR monitoring must be based on an easy, simplified and comprehensible format that outlines clearly and point by point the actions to be accomplished. This action-based format should contain:

1) Pertinent data of the patient (name, age, sex, weight and height).
2) Service information (name of service and clinical file number).
3) Disease information (diagnosis, heart rate, temperature, arterial pressure and serum creatinine).
4) Medication information (name of drug or drugs and daily doses)
5) ADR suspected drug (name, dose and administration frequency).
6) ADRs observed.
7) Affected systems and related symptoms.
8) Actions against ADRs and the outcomes.
9) Possible causes of the observed ADRs.

1. Patient´s data
Name of patient ____________ age ________ gender ______ weight ________ height ______
2. Service information: Name of service: _____________ No. of clinical file: _____________
3. Disease information
Diagnosis: ___________________ heart rate: _____________ temperature: _______________ arterial pressure: ________________ serum creatinine: _______________.
4. Medication information Drug: ____________________ doses/day: ____________________.
5. ADR suspected drug information: doses/administered _____________________________
6. ADRs observed.
Instructions: -complete the following paragraphs with: yes (tick good), or no (x) (do not leave any space blank). If you have any doubt, contact pharmacology laboratory staff.
Tachycardia ________ bradycardia _________ anorexy ________ nauseas ________ diarrhea _______ vomiting _______ constipation _______ colic _______ acidity _______ abdominal distention ______ oral dryness ______ urinary retention ______ dizziness ________ skin rash ______ somnolence __________ hypoxy ________ blurred vision ________ confusion ________ weakness ________ delirium _______ hypothermia ________ fever ________ insomnium ________ allucinations ________ palpitations ______ edema ______ arrhythmia ______ sedation ____________ respiratory depression ______ sedation ________ agitation ________ AV block ________ hypoactivity ________ convulsions ______ coma _______ pain ______ headache ______ muscular ______ extremities ______ renal ______ chest ______ stomach ache______

Figure 1. (Continued)

7. Affected systems and related symptoms: Gastrointestinal ________ hematological ________ dermatological ________ sensorial________ CNS ______ autonomous ___________ respiratory ____________ genitourinary __________ cardiovascular ____________ teratogenic _______ immunologic ______ others
8. Actions against ADRs and the outcomes :
Required drug suspension ______________ required change of doses _____________ disappeared on changing the drug ___________ time of disappearance: at ________ hours.
9. Possible cause of the observed ADRs: Adverse effects _________ overdose ________ intolerance _____ idiosyncrasy ______ drug interaction________ added pathology ________ renal insufficiency ______ hypersensitivity _______ hepatic insufficiency _____
10. Observations and comments of the treating medical staff(s) ____
11. Reporting the incidence to the pharmacology department:___________ Date ______

Figure 1. Format applied for pharmacovigelance program.

10) Observations and comments of the treating medical staff(s) and
11) Reporting the incidence to the Pharmacology department (Figure 1).

It is important to understand that any assumption of ADR for any drug is conclusive only when the reactions reported for that drug, the response patterns, disease-drug interactions and drug-drug interactions are investigated in the relevant literature [3, 4]. If the results of the bibliographical investigation match the profile of ADRs for the drug then, the above ADR monitoring actions should be implemented. Moreover, it is important to assess the severity of the patient and this can be done by stopping the administration of the suspected ADR-producing drug and observing the patient´s response. If such response is favorable, an alternative treatment should be given to the patient. Nevertheless, if the response is tolerable, drug administration can continue, but at a different dose to observe the participation of other drugs jointly administered with the ADR-producing drug.

It is important to point out that as easy as this program seems, ADR monitoring through PV is not an easy task. Its set-off and effectiveness require convincing and motivating the medical staff and the nurses, the first in line in the detection of the undesirable effects of drugs for their closer contact with patients.

It is needless to say that ADR monitoring through efficient PV program is fraught with meritorious advantages such as improvement in the treatment schemes. As the saying goes "experience is the best teacher" and this is true of drug management where a safe use is based on acquired experience and consequently the achievement of a better quality of attention to the patients. This is amply discussed in previous reports [5-8]. Since the onset of the PV program in this hospital, 141 ADRs were reported with most of them being provoked by intoxication due to elevated drug dose and with the discovery that the principal causes of ADRs are the oncologic drugs.

PHARMACOEPIDEMIOLOGY

The drugs prescribed and consumed by a population are generally conditioned by a series of factors among which socio-economic, genetic-hereditary, hygienic and cultural characteristics can be mentioned. The drug market is guided by patterns of drug consumption. Drug availability responds to these patterns, thus, studies on drug prescription and consumption profiles are necessary.

Results of PE investigations suggest therapeutic resources and permit the deduction of individual treatments, mainly by considering the age of patients [9, 10].

At the pediatrics hospital, the patients present particular features. A great number of them who seek consultation show some degree of malnutrition, and most families depend only on a single income source, usually produced by the fathers and sometimes by the mothers. Only on occasions do both parents participate in the family bread winning.

Genetic features have recently been investigated with the unfortunate finding that the predominant metabolic profiles have yet not been characterized. However, the pharmacokinetic behavior due to biological issues has been described for various drugs such as salicylates and some antibiotics.

The socio-economic status has a direct link with the hygienic conditions in determining the frequent ailments which a population suffers. Issues such as hand washing and consumption of clean food, just to mention a few, are directly related to hygienic habits and economic status. There are also cultural issues of the patients' families that weigh on the decision of whether health attention, time investment and expenses should be a priority, and on the healing method to adopt.

For instance, taking non-professional recommendations, searching for and using idiosyncratic remedies such as herbalists, ritual cleansing, spells, etc. [11].

Objectives of PE Program

An efficient and effective PE program must aim at:

1) Achieving the required expertize to control the most frequently used drugs, both in clinical services and in the entire hospital.
2) Determining all the variables that describe drug consumption profile in a population, based on the main diagnoses of the patients attendants data in the hospital.
3) Developing the needed expertize capable of preparing at therapeutic drug formula based on the characteristics of the attended population in order to optimize the proper use of drugs.

Procedure

APE inquiry depends on the service in which the drug consumption profiles is investigated. Such inquiry must be based on a format (Figure 2), which does not vary much among the services and must contain the following sections:

1) Patients identification.
2) Gestation and birth information.
3) Diagnoses on admission.
4) Added diagnoses in the ward.
5) Discharge information
6) Diagnoses at discharge and
7) Medication information.

1. Identification. Name: __________________ Dept and/or service __________________

Place of origin ______________ Reg. no. __________ age (months/days) ____________ Date of admission _______________ Gender ___________ actual weight __________ actual height (cm) ______________

2. Gestation and birth information. Gesta ____________ Birth weight _____________ weeks of gestation _____________ Birth height __________ Date of birth ____________

3. Diagnoses on admission:
1.____
2.____
3.____
4.____
5.____

Figure 2. (Continued)

4. Added diagnoses during admission:
1. ______________________________ Date ________________________
2. ______________________________ Date ________________________
3. ______________________________ Date ________________________
4. ______________________________ Date ________________________

5. Discharge information. Date ___________ weight _________ height _____________

6. Diagnoses on discharge
1.____
2.____
3.____

7. Medication information

Drug	Commencement date	Ending date	doses (mg/kg/ day)	dose interval	clinical effects*

* associated with the administration of medication.
Elaborated by: Name _________ Professional license number ______
Signature: ________

Figure 2. Format applied for pharmacoepidemiology program.

The origin of all the drugs administered during the hospital stay must be investigated, i.e., if they were acquired directly from the pharmacy or somewhere else. Although these data are descriptively analyzed, they are subsequently compared to drug consumption patterns in other places with similar conditions. The conclusions of each study are published among physicians, since this could help to improve future prescription schemes. This has been found helpful in the area of antibiotics and chemotherapeutic agent prescription, since effectiveness depends on their proper use due to the high prevailing rates of resistance [12, 13]. As in other activities, the respective format is a necessary instrument for the development of this activity. However, depending on the site of study or duration, there may be some modifications in the format. For instance, in some studies in rural communities, few different questions aimed at obtaining information on a specific environment were included in the format [11]. The authors have studied 670 patients consisting of males (54.17%) and females (45.82%) with ages oscillating from 16.2 days to 14.8 years and weight from 3.4 to 56.3kg. The authors found that the most commonly prescribed drugs were antibiotics in 29%, followed by gastrointestinal medicaments in 23.5%. Two to four drugs per patient were prescribed, which was in agreement with the previously published data [13].

DISCUSSION

PV and PE are important tools that open doors to a better drug prescription scheme and guide towards a better drug use in patients in all health institutes. An effective PV and PE must follow a line of actions in a well-defined procedure with objectives. When these lines of actions are meticulously followed, beneficial results such as the knowledge of ADR-producing drugs and their avoidance, the nature of their adverse effects and effective way to tackle them when they occur are obtained. Moreover, it enables health centers to keep track of drugs mostly consumed, take note of disease-related drug resistance, minimize polypharmacy and above all optimize resources. Also, they ensure a constant flow of information on the profile of drug products currently used by a center, information that could enrich the database of the central agency of PE for the benefit of all health staffs.

At the National Institute of Pediatrics of Mexico, the experiences acquired on PV and PE applications have yielded important results. Pharmacology Department, which is in charge of PV and PE in the Institute has outlined the procedures, objectives and definitions of all the activities performed. Through these activities, the service has observed an increase in the incidence of ADR in a larger number of drug prescriptions, mainly in patients who took more than two drugs simultaneously, which is very common [2]. In the light of this, the department has issued important recommendations based on individualizing therapies among patients, reducing the polypharmacy that gives rise to drug interactions and adopts measures to prevent or diminish these effects when they occur. The ADR-offsetting measures include suspension of all drugs to investigate the ADR-producing drug and in case the effect is due to overdose, to check the plasmatic drug levels [14] and reduce the drug dosage [3].

In terms of PE, the department found that drugs used for the treatment of infectious diseases rank first as the most commonly prescribed and consumed drugs in the Institute followed by gastrointestinal disease drugs and nutritional complements in the third place [13]. The frequent use of antibiotics is due to their administration before, during and after any surgical procedure, as well as for the treatment of infectious diseases. It recognized the importance of establishing services such as PV and PE to help control drug usage. Since PV and PE activities were initiated in the hospital, they have contributed to a more adequate use of drugs in children. The development and implementation of PV and PE at our hospital has enriched both the clinical practice and our staff's work, since it has consistently forced us to seek better options for the adequate use of drugs in children. As the first conclusion of our PV and PE activities, we can recommend that, if polytherapy is not necessary, it must be avoided. Through PE activities, drug consumption can be optimally planned in the hospital, with the intention of acquiring only those medicaments to be used, avoiding waste and caring for the hospital economy. Finally, the present guide can be adopted at hospitals interested in initiating PV and PE.

REFERENCES

[1] Carnovale, C., Brusadelli, T., Zuccotti, G., Beretta, S., Sullo, M. G., Capuano, A., Rossi, F., Moschini, M., Mugelli, A., Vannacci, A., Laterza, M., Clementi, E., Radice, S.; MEAP Group. The importance of monitoring adverse drug reactions in pediatric patients: the results of a national surveillance program in Italy. *Expert Opin. Drug Saf.*, 2014; 13 Suppl. 1:S1-8.

[2] Al Dweik, R., Stacey, D., Kohen, D., Yaya, S. Factors affecting patient reporting of adverse drug reactions: a systematic review. *Br. J. Clin. Pharmacol.*, 2017;83:875-883.

[3] Tanti, A., Serracino-Inglott, A., Borg, J. J. Designing a national combined reporting form for adverse drug reactions and medication errors. *East Mediterr. Health J.*, 2015; 21:246-55.

[4] Yu, Y. M., Lee, E. Enhanced knowledge of spontaneous reporting with structured educational programs in Korean community pharmacists: a cross-sectional study. *BMC Med. Educ.*, 2017; 17:95.

[5] Varallo, F. R., Planeta, C. S., Mastroianni, P. C. Effectiveness of pharmacovigilance: multifaceted educational intervention related to the knowledge, skills and attitudes of multidisciplinary hospital staff. *Clinics.* (Sao Paulo), 2017; 72:51-57.

[6] Pathak, A. K. 1., Kumar, M2., Dokania, S3., Mohan, L4., Dikshit, H5. A retrospective analysis of reporting of adverse drug reactions in a tertiary care teaching hospital: One year survey. *J Clin. Diagn. Res.*, 2016; 10:FC01-4.

[7] Hutton, B., Kanji, S., McDonald, E., Yazdi, F., Wolfe, D., Thavorn, K., Pepper, S., Chapman, L., Skidmore, B., Moher, D. Incidence, causes, and consequences of preventable adverse drug events: protocol for an overview of reviews. *Syst. Rev.*, 2016; 5:209.

[8] Perez-Guille, G., Guille-Perez, A., Larios-Mejia, C., Camacho-Vieyra, A., Juarez-Olguın, H., Lares Asseff, I. Las directrices que rigen la terapeutica farmacologica en el recien nacido. [The guidelines governing pharmacological therapeutics in the newborn] *Perinatol Reprod Hum.* 2000; 14:22–31.

[9] Naeeni, M. M., Jafari, S., Fouladgar, M., Heidari, K., Farajzadegan, Z., Fakhri, M., Karami, P., Omidi, R. Nutritional knowledge, practice, and dietary habits among school children and adolescents. *Int. J. Prev. Med.,* 2014; 5 (Suppl. 2):S171-8.

[10] Perez-Guille, G., Camacho-Vieyra, A., Toledo-Lopez, A., Guille-Perez, A., Flores-Perez, J., Juarez-Olguın, H. Patterns of drug consumption in relation with diseases in elderly patients of Mexico. *J. Pharm. Pharmaceut. Sci.,* 2001; 4:177-184.

[11] Juarez-Olguın, H., Chico-Aldama, P., Hidalgo Felipede Jesus, Perez-Guille, G., Camacho-Vieyra, A., Guille-Perez, A. Patterns of drug prescription and consumption in a rural community of Morelos Mexico. *J. Pharm. Pract. Res.,* 2003; 33:330.

[12] Bekker, A., Schaaf, H. S., Draper, H. R., van der Laan, L., Murray, S., Wiesner, L., Donald, P. R., McIlleron, H. M., Hesseling, A. C. Pharmacokinetics of rifampin, isoniazid, pyrazinamide, and ethambutol in infants dosed according to revised who-recommended treatment guidelines. *Antimicrob. Agents Chemother.*, 2016; 60: 2171-9.

[13] de Bie, S., Kaguelidou, F., Verhamme, K. M., De Ridder, M., Picelli, G., Straus, S. M., Giaquinto, C., Stricker, B. H., Bielicki, J., Sharland, M., Sturkenboom, M. C.; ARPEC study. Using prescription patterns in primary care to derive new quality indicators for childhood community antibiotic prescribing. *Pediatr. Infect. Dis. J.*, 2016 Dec.; 35(12):1317-1323.

[14] Juarez-Olguın, H., Flores-Perez, J., Lares-Asseff, I., Flores-Perez, C., Perez-Guille, G., Camacho-Vieyra, A., Guille-Perez, A., Calderon-Guzman, D. Medication-related services in a Mexican pediatric hospital. *Am. J. Health Syst. Pharm.*, 2004; 61:2311–2312.

In: The Optimization of Drug Prescribing … ISBN: 978-1-53612-263-3
Editor: Hugo Juarez Olguin

Chapter 10

UNINTENTIONAL DRUG POISONING IN THE PEDIATRIC POPULATION

Hugo Juarez Olguín[1,2,*], Carmen Flores Pérez[1,2] and Janett Flores Pérez[1]

[1]Laboratorio de Farmacología, Instituto Nacional de Pediatría, Mexico City, Mexico

[2]Departamento de Farmacología, Facultad de Medicina, Universidad Nacional Autónoma de México. Mexico

ABSTRACT

More than 70% of acute pediatric poisoning is caused by medications. The age group sat the greatest risk of this incident are those between 2 to 5 years and 14 to 18 years, although in this last group, drug ingestion is usually intentional. The purpose of this chapter is to describe the frequency of unintentional drug poisoning in pediatric population, and to review the treatment procedures applied in specific cases. In most of the cases, poisoning is confirmed by determining the plasma concentration of the drug. The most frequent cases of drug poisoning

* Corresponding Author Email: juarezol@yahoo.com

were due to the ingestion of drugs like analgesics mainly acetylsalicylic acid and acetaminophen, antiepileptics, anxiolytics and in lesser proportion other drugs. With the exception of accidental ingestion of drugs, drug poisoning in pediatric population is mainly due to dosing error. Self-medication in this population is unlikely for their age. In most of the cases of unintentional drug poisoning seen in this series, the duration of hospitalization did not exceed 24 hours and no death was registered. Dosing error should be a topic of a major concern for hospitals since this error has been found to be the principal cause of unintentional drug poisoning in infants and young children.

INTRODUCTION

More than 70% of acute pediatric poisoning is caused by medications [1]. According to the Poison Control Centers (AAPCC), children under 6 years of age are accidentally exposed to medication for their characteristic nature of putting practically everything they lay hands on into their mouth [2]. The age group sat the greatest risk of drug poisoning are those between 2 to 5 and 14 to 18 years old although in this last group, drug ingestion is usually intentional [3]. Analgesics like acetylsalicylic acid and acetaminophen have been reported to be among the drugs commonly used in the pediatric population that usually cause poisoning [4]. Since these drugs are not controlled, they are found in most drug stores. Hence, they are available to the general public. Other studies have reported drug poisoning with antiepileptics like phenytoin, carbamazepine, phenobarbital and valproic acid [5]. Drug poisoning has also been seen with antihistamines such as chlorphenamine, diphenhydramine and astemizole [6, 7]. Similarly, digoxin has been found to provoke many poisoning. The onset of digoxin poisoning begins at 3.0 ng/Ml and because of its narrow margin between the therapeutic and toxic plasma concentrations [8], it is easy to exceed this levels in the patients.

To study the drugs that most frequently produce poisoning in pediatric population, it is important to consider the pharmacokinetic factors and the dynamic physiological characteristics of this age. It is also essential to involve all clinicians in the situation in order to detect such events on time, register them and offer adequate intervention. Unfortunately, there are few studies on this topic not only in pediatrics but also in the general population. The objectives of this report were to determine the frequency of unintentional drug poisoning in pediatric population and to review the treatment procedures applied in specific cases.

EXAMPLE OF UNINTENTIONAL DRUG POISONING

The report is based on a study performed at the National Pediatrics Institute (INP, for its initials in Spanish). INP is a tertiary care hospital and a major medical center for children in Mexico. The institute has about 8,000 in patients and every year it conducts approximately 200,000 consultations, performs more than 6,000 surgical interventions, and carries out 500,000 laboratory tests. A significant percentage of the patients have chronic and complex diseases, and a small number are admitted due to acute conditions. Many of the patients that seek for medical attention in the hospital require multiple treatments, hospitalization, and subsequent follow-up, some of which are long term. Admissions in the hospital are usually for pediatric patients who require specialist attention, including patients with suspicion of poisoning.

Unintentional drug poisoning (UDP) at National Pediatric Institute was retrospectively reviewed. UDP is defined as an accidental intake of drug due to a mistake in dosage. UDP cases in the hospital were obtained from a data base of the Clinical Record Department. The International Statistical Classification of Diseases and Related Health Problems [9] criteria were applied to determine cases of UDP in the clinical records. In all confirmed UDP cases, information such as patient's demographic data (age and gender), the poisoning-causing drugs, the treatment given for the poison and the severity of the injury were compiled (*see* Table 1). Plasma concentrations found in the files were registered. Results were analyzed based on the frequency of each of the poisoning-causing drugs in the children.

Table 1. Treatment measures used for unintentional drug poisoning[a]

Drug class	Treatment	% of poisoned children
Analgesics	Gastriclavage Activated charcoal	26.5% (37cases)
	N-acetylcysteine[b]	15.8% (22cases)
Anxiolytic agents	Gastriclavage Activated charcoal	10% (14 cases)
	Flumazenil[c]	7.9% (11 cases)
Antiepileptic agents	Therapeutic Drug Monitoring Neurological monitoring	23% (32 cases)
Positive inotropic agents	Electrocardiographic monitoring Hemodynamic monitoring	14% (20 cases)

[a] In 33/139 cases, the use of a specific antidote in the children was necessary and the plasma concentrations of the drug were measured;

[b] drug used for the cases of acetaminophen poisoning;

[c] drug used for the cases of diazepam poisoning.

Data Analysis

One hundred and thirty nine (139) clinical records, with diagnosis of unintentional drug poisoning (UDP) determined based on the criteria of the International Statistical Classification of Diseases and Related Health Problems, were reviewed. Of the pediatric population found to have suffered UDP, 122 were healthy children while in the rest, the underlying diseases were epilepsy (12 cases) and congestive heart failure (5 cases).

The age range for the cases of poisoning was from 7 days to13 years of age (median 2 years). The gender distribution was 62 females and 77 males. Of all the cases, only in 21children was UDP caused by self- administered accidental over dose.

On analyzing the ages of the patients, it was found that children younger than 2 years old, representing 49.6% of the studied population, were the most vulnerable to drug poisoning followed by children between 2 and 5 years of age with 38.1% and those between 6 and13 years of age with 12.2%. Therapeutic drug monitoring was carried out in 33cases (23.7%) by measurement of specific drug plasma concentrations.

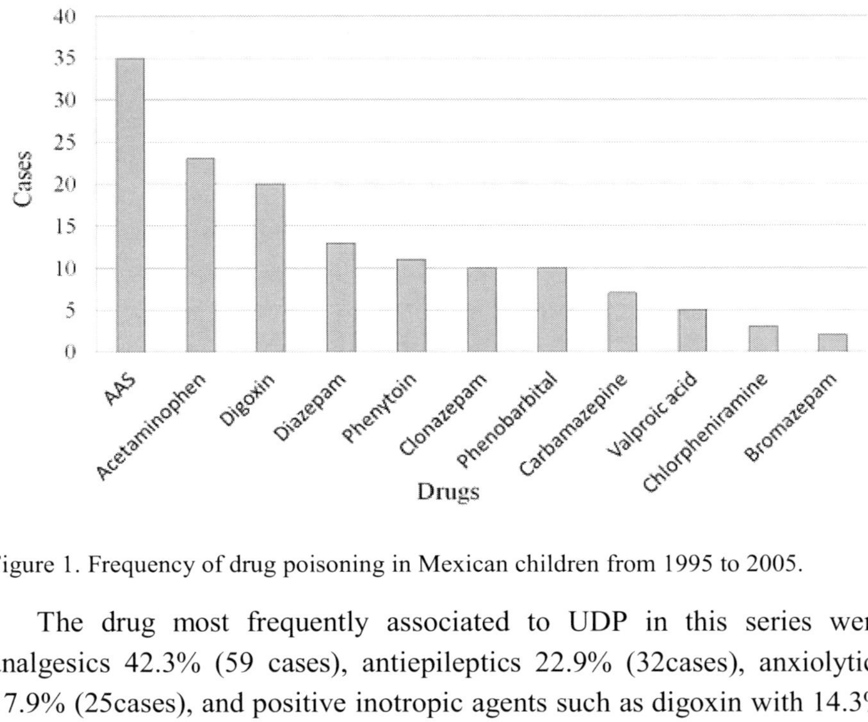

Figure 1. Frequency of drug poisoning in Mexican children from 1995 to 2005.

The drug most frequently associated to UDP in this series were analgesics 42.3% (59 cases), antiepileptics 22.9% (32cases), anxiolytics 17.9% (25cases), and positive inotropic agents such as digoxin with 14.3% (20 cases). In the cases of analgesics, acetylsalicylic acid accounted for 35 cases and acetaminophen for 24 cases. Of the 24 cases of acetaminophen, 15 were patients under 1 year of age, 6 were 2-5 years old and 3 patients were older than 6 years. With regard to the antiepileptics, phenytoin accounted for 11 cases, phenobarbital 10 cases, carbamazepine 6 cases and valproic acid 5 cases. For anxiolytic drugs, diazepam was responsible for 13 cases, clonazepam for 10 cases and bromazepam for 2 cases. These data are shown graphically in Figure 1.

TREATMENTS EMPLOYED IN THE CASES

Treatments used in the cases were non-pharmacological and pharmacological. In the choice of the treatment type, the culprit drug, the severity of the poisoning and the clinical manifestations were considered. In general and with previous assessment of the culprit drug ingestion route, measures taken for the treatment were as follows: gastric lavage and administration of activated charcoal in 87 cases of analgesic, anxiolytic and antihistamine poisonings; administration of N-acetylcysteine as an antidote before and after hepatic assessment to 22 cases of acetaminophen poisoning confirmed by plasma concentration determination; neurological and therapeutic drug monitoring to 32 patients with antiepileptic drug poisoning confirmed by clinical diagnosis; constant electrocardiographic and close hemodynamic monitoring for 20 cases of digoxin poisoning; and flumazenil antidote to 11 children with diazepam poisoning. Table 1 summarizes the information on treatment measures that are commonly used in pediatric population for drug poisoning.

EXPECTATIONS AND CONCLUSION

The results of the in this series are similar to what were previously reported[10], where analgesics were found to be the most frequent drug involved in accidental poisoning with acetylsalicylic acid ranking first followed by acetaminophen [11, 12]. Unfortunately, these two analgesics are sold over-the-counter.

The children in this series were clinically assessed using the Glasgow and ABC resuscitation scales to determine their states of consciousness.

122 of the children were healthy and did not require drugs to treat any disease, thereby indicating that the poisoning was unintentional. Also, poisoning due to self-medication is not likely because of the age of the children hence, the drugs that provoke the poisoning were probably unintentionally ingested.

Coupled with unintentional ingestion is the lack of infant dosages in many drugs. Most of the drugs used in treating pediatric patients are only available in adult formulations. So, to apply them to the children requires dose calculation or modification and most of the time, this action is fraught with errors that may lead to poisoning. At National Pediatric Institute, Mexico City, all the cases of poisoning were reported as unintentional for the fact that they originated from errors in dose modification.

Another factor that might have contributed to drug poisoning in this population is physiological factors. At early ages, physiological changes due to growth and development are still present, thus the body is sometimes incapable of metabolizing and eliminating drugs adequately. In this series however, none of the cases required more than 24hours of hospitalization, and none of the analyzed patients died due to poisoning. In the light of the above results, we recommend that in young children, extreme care must be taken in the use of drugs such as analgesics, antiepileptics and anxiolytics since they constitute the most frequent cause of unintentional drug poisoning in infants.

REFERENCES

[1] Mináriková, M., Fojtikova, V., Vyskočilová, E., Sedláček, J., Šikut, M., Borek-Dohalska, L., Stiborová, M., Martinkova, M. The capacity and effectiveness of diosmectite and charcoal in trapping the compounds causing the most frequent intoxications in acute medicine: A comparative study. *Environ. Toxicol. Pharmacol.* 2017 Jun; 52:214-220.

[2] Litovitz, T. L., Klein-Schwartz, W., Caravati, E. M. Annual report of the American Association of Poison Control Centers Toxic Exposure Surveillance System. *Am. J. Emerg. Med.* 1999; 17: 435-87.

[3] Lifshitz, M., Gavrilov, V. Acute poisoning in children. *Israel Med. Assoc. J.* 2000; 2:504-6.

[4] Shannon, M. Ingestion of toxic substances by children. *N. Eng. J. Med.* 2000; 342: 186-91.

[5] Riordan, M., Rylance, G., Berry, K. Poisoning in children 5: Rare and dangerous poisons. *Arch. Dis. Child* 2002; 87: 407-10.

[6] Acosta-Materán, C., Díaz-Oliva, E., Fernández-Rodríguez, D., Hernández-Afonso, J. QT interval prolongation and torsade de pointes: Synergistic effect of flecainide and H1 receptor antagonists. *J. Pharmacol. Pharmac.* other. 2016 Apr-Jun; 7(2):102-5.

[7] Tilelli, J. A., Smith, K. M., Pettignano, R. Life-threatening bradyarrhythmia after massive azithromycin overdose. *Pharmacotherapy*. 2006 Jan; 26 (1):147-50.

[8] Tsuruoka, S., Osono, E., Nishiki, K., Kawaguchi, A., Arai, T., Furuyoshi, S., Saito, T., Takata, S., Sugimoto, K., Kurihara, S., Fujimura, A. Removal of digoxin by column for specific adsorption of beta (2)-microglobulin: a potential use for digoxin intoxication. *Clin. Pharmacol. Ther.* 2001 Jun; 69(6):422-30.

[9] *International Statistical Classification of Diseases and Related Health Problems.* Tenth Revision. Pan American Health Organization. World Health Organization 1995. Version for 2007 http:// www. who.int/classifications/apps/icd/icd10online.

[10] Juurlink, D. N., Gosselin, S., Kielstein, J. T., Ghannoum, M., Lavergne, V., Nolin, T. D., Hoffman, R. S.; EXTRIP Workgroup. Extracorporeal Treatment for Salicylate Poisoning: Systematic Review and Recommendations. From the EXTRIP Workgroup. *Ann. Emerg. Med.* 2015 Aug; 66(2):165-81.

[11] Stewart, J. E., Haslam, A. K., Puig, J. Pathology in Practice. Acetaminophen (paracetamol) toxicosis. *J. Am. Vet. Med. Assoc.* 2016 May 1; 248(9):1009-11.

[12] Flores Perez, C., Juarez Olguin, H., Chavez Pacheco, J. l., Flores Perez, J. Validation of acetaminofen and its metabolite by a HPLC method applied for children studies. *Biomedical Chromatography* 25: 760-766, 2011.

In: The Optimization of Drug Prescribing … ISBN: 978-1-53612-263-3
Editor: Hugo Juarez Olguin

Chapter 11

SUICIDAL ATTEMPTS BY CONSUMPTION OF DRUGS IN CHILDREN

Mónica Punzo Soto, Carmen Flores Pérez* and Mayra Santillán García
Laboratorio de Farmacología, Instituto Nacional de Pediatría, Mexico City, Mexico

ABSTRACT

Suicide is presently a serious health problem that is seen in different age groups. Most of the children and adolescents that commit suicide have some kind of psychiatric illness and sometimes, small predictors of suicidal ideation are overlooked. Suicidal behavior in children is a delicate topic because in them, it is difficult to predict this behavior.

This chapter intends to invite pediatricians, health professionals and authorities to implement actions of alertness to detect factors that could lead to suicide in order to reduce its figures and incidences, especially in pediatric patients.

*Corresponding Author Email: carmenfloresp@hotmail.com

Introduction

Suicide is a complex behavior with biological, psychological and social causes, with predisposing family factors such as domestic violence, psychiatric disorders, and alcohol abuse by parents [1]. Suicide attempt, defined as "thoughts and/or actions that if fully carried out may lead to serious self-injury or death" [2], is a tragedy that affects families, communities and countries, and it is considered as a serious public health problem which can occur at any age. As of 2015, this problem is regarded as the second cause of death in the age group of 15 to 29 years [3]. The annual record by WHO puts the toll at 800,000 and 78% of the cases is found in low-income countries. The most vulnerable groups are principally those who are object of discrimination as refugees, migrants and indigenous communities among others. Suicidal behavior in children is a subject of great concern because of their cognitive immaturity to express suicidal feelings. In the past, it was believed that children were not capable of suicidal ideation, planning and much less the execution of such acts. However, several studies have shown that children are capable of successfully committing suicide [2]. A number of risk factors associated with suicide have been identified and the most important individual factor is a frustrated attempt to commit suicide [3]. Nevertheless, the timely identification of patients at risk as well as specific interventions is of vital importance since it is totally a preventable cause of death. In 2014, the first worldwide report on suicide was published by WHO in a paper titled "Prevention of Suicide: A Global Imperative", which aims to sensitize the world population on the problem of suicide. In the mental health plan 2013–2020, WHO member states committed themselves to achieving the global goal of reducing national suicide rate by 10% in 2020.

Risk Factors

Children with suicidal ideation are usually people with antisocial behavior and in those from 5 to 14 years of age, it is more frequent in boys than in girls with a proportion of 3:1 [4]. It has been reported that up to 40% of suicide cases in children are preceded by previous suicide attempt and that in one-third of the cases a first or second-degree relative with a history of suicidal behavior is identified [1] and because the children do not completely understand the consequences of suicidal act, they try to imitate it.

The presence of psychiatric disease in child has also been associated with suicide ideation and depression is the most identified in these children. In serotoninergic system, the levels of serotonin and its metabolite (5-hydroxyindolacetic acid) are in lower concentrations in suicidal patients. This system regulates the impulsiveness, aggressiveness and mood. In patients with suicidal behavior, the three factors above are altered [5] and this can be manifested by the patient as unsatisfactory and inconformity with their life style.

The main risk factors associated are: previous suicide attempt (risk rises 6 times), psychiatric disorder (bulimia 48%, depression or anxiety crisis 34%, defiant opposition disorder 33%, combined ADHD 22%, anorexia 22%, autism 18%, intellectual disability 17%, and inattentive-ADHD type), excessive worry for death, history of family suicidal behavior or psychiatric illness (mainly of the mother), divorced parents and history of family abuse [6,7].

In the study of Dickerson et al, suicidal ideation was correlated with behavioral eating disorder using multiple psychological and demographical sleep variables. In the study, 90 children with ages ranging from 7 to 18 years were enrolled. The main finding was that suicidal ideation was more frequent in children with nervous bulimia (43%) than in children with nervous anorexia (20%). All children with nervous bulimia tried to commit suicide while only 3% of the children with nervous anorexia did. The correlates of attempts were nervous bulimia, self-induced vomits, nightmares and physical or sexual abuse [8].

Bullying is a systematic power abuse and is defined as aggressive behavior or intentional damage carried out repeatedly by peers and which implies imbalance in power [9]. Currently, the presence of bullying has been observed as a risk factor for suicide. Dickerson et al., presented the first study in patients of 6-18 years of age where the frequencies of suicidal behavior were compared in 5 groups: intimidation, bully, victim, bully/victim and none and concluded that harassment forms part of an independent risk factor and demonstrated that the patients exposed to harassment are more prone to problems of sadness and greater tendency towards suicidal ideations [10].

With this, we want to demonstrate that eating, behavioral and school disorders play a vital role in suicide-predicating behavior, which should not be ignored as physicians and health professionals.

METHODS OF SUICIDE

There is poor availability and quality of data on suicide. In children, the information is usually misclassified for the fact that it is not always easy to decipher if the death is caused by accident or other cause because until now, it is still difficult for people to believe that a child (especially under 12 years) is capable of devising, planning and executing suicide acts. Hence, the existence of information to elaborate adequate prevention strategies is indispensable.

Based on current available information, we can conclude that the most common methods are: self-poisoning by medication, where the drugs of highest intake are sedatives [4], analgesics/antidepressants [8] and pesticides [3] normally common in children of 6 to 10 years; hanging; self-immolation; jumping from high places or down stairs; stepping in front of a moving vehicle; intentional drowning; cutting and medication overdose [4].

A retrospective cohort involving a follow-up of 40 patients who intentionally ingested a drug for the sole purpose of committing suicide revealed that the most frequent medications were analgesics (paracetamol, acetylsalicylic acid, naproxen and tramadol) in 18 patients; antidepressants (alprazolam, diazepam and clonazepam) in 10; antiepileptics (carbamazepine) in 5, antibiotics (ampicillin, cloramphenicol and amoxicillin) in 4 patients, antipsychotics (trifuoperazine and haloperidol) in 2 and hypoglycemic agents (glibenclamide and metformin) in 1 patient (Figure 1).

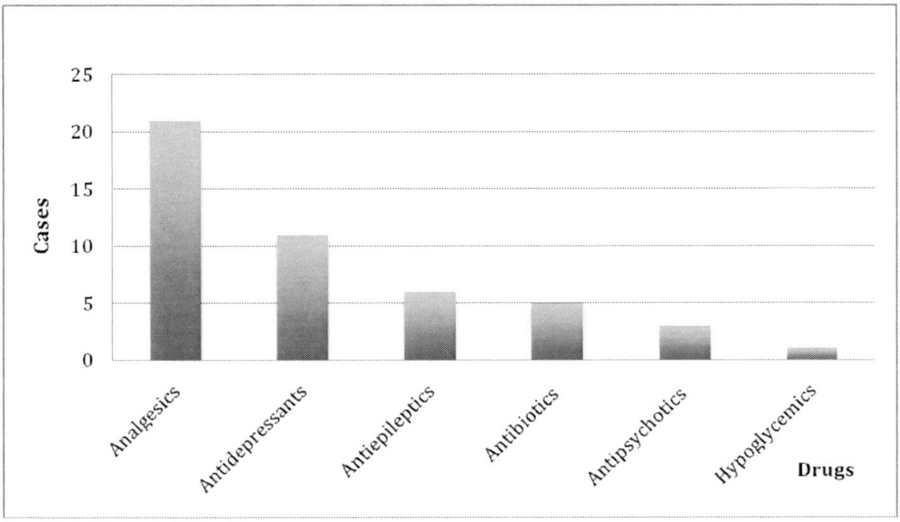

Figure 1. Drug frequency in attempted suicide.

PREVENTION

The increase in the incidence of suicide in children shows that the risk factors, motivations as well as the methods used to perpetrate suicide are increasing. This may be owed to the fact that children as well as adolescents are so susceptible to commit suicide when they are exposed to risk factors. The society and the health personnel should be properly educated to identify alert data [4]. The problem we face in this regard is that children usually show less data of alarm and the few we can identify are difficult to predict. The parents usually underestimate the possibility of suicidal commission of the children and for them as well as for the physicians it is easy to confuse a suicidal attempt with "accidents" hence, it is important to remember that in the face of any alarm data, attention should be placed on the child. Such a child must be kept in a place devoid of lethal substances and must not be left alone.

Recommendations on the Topic

From the points previously exposed and discussed in this work, we can identify that suicide is a complex problem that demands urgent populational preventive measures, since it is totally preventable. These preventive measures can be carried out through the coordination of multiple sectors of the society such as the health sector, ministry of education, etc. The most important is to identify patients that are susceptible.

The first principle for the assessment of suicide is to take seriously the ideation. Sarcasm and jokes as well as challenging or devaluing the person who reveal this kind of ideas must be scrupulously avoided.

The second principle is to assess the individual within biopsychosocial framework [5].

The most important measures that must be taken into account are:

- Restriction of all access to means of suicide e.g., drugs, pesticides, guns, etc.
- Responsible information
- Policies directed in reducing harmful alcohol consumption
- Timely identification, treatment and personal attention to mental health problems and abuse of substances as well as chronic pain.
- Training the health personnel in the evaluation and management of suicidal behavior.
- Fellow-up of people with history of suicidal attempt as well as providing community support.

References

[1] Flores, P. J., Juárez, O. H., Flores, P. C., Rivera, E. L. Suicide attempts by ingestion of drugs in adolescents in Mexico. *J. Clinic. Toxicol.* 2011; S1:005.

[2] Juárez, O. H., Barranco, G. M., Flores, P. J., Acosta, B. M., Flores, P. C. Frequency of suicide attempts by ingestion of drugs seen at a tertiary care pediatric hospital in Mexico. *J. Popul. Ther. Clin. Pharmacol.* 2011; 18:161-165.

[3] World Health Organization. *Preventing suicide: A global imperative.* World Health Organization 2014.

[4] Tishler, L., Reiss, N., Rhodes, A. Suicidal behavior in children younger than twelve: a diagnostic challenge for emergency department personnel. *Acad. Emerg. Med.* 2007; 14:810–818.

[5] Nelson Kliegman, M., Jenson, B., Staton, F., Chapter 26. Suicidio e intento de suicidio. In: Boris W, Dalton R. *Tratado de pediatría Nelson*, (2012) 19e. [Chapter 26. Suicide and attempted suicide]

[6] Dickerson, M., Calhoun, S., Baweja, R. Suicide ideation and attempts in children with psychiatric disorders and typical development. *Crisis*, 2015; 36:55-60.

[7] Toussig, H., Harpin, S., Maguire, S. Suicidality among preadolescent maltreated children in foster care. *Child Matreat*. 2014; 19:17-26.

[8] Dickerson, M., Fernandez, M., Baweja, R. Correlates of suicide ideation and attempts in children and adolescents with eating disorders. *Eat. Disord.* 2014; 22:352-66.

[9] Wolke, D., Lereya, S. Long-term effects of bullying. *Arch. Dis. Child* 2015; 100:879-85.

[10] Dickerson, M., Bawejar, R., Calhoun, S. Suicide ideation and attempts and bullying in children and adolescents: psychiatric and general population samples. *Crisis* 2014; 35:301-9.

INDEX

A

absorption, ix, 5, 6, 12, 19, 27, 29, 31, 35, 36, 37, 39, 40, 41, 43, 44, 49, 75, 76, 77, 78, 79, 80, 81, 82, 86, 98, 99, 100, 101, 102, 137, 139, 143, 146, 148, 168, 169, 174, 185
accidental over dose, 207
accidents, 63, 64, 217
acetaminophen, xii, 46, 81, 84, 85, 102, 204, 206, 207, 208, 210, 211
acetylsalicylic acid, xii, 204, 207, 208, 216
acid, xii, 45, 49, 62, 79, 80, 84, 86, 97, 101, 102, 103, 105, 108, 110, 145, 176, 204, 207, 208, 215, 216
acidity, 43, 78, 100, 193
adipose tissue, 83
administration, ix, xi, 2, 10, 11, 12, 14, 16, 19, 27, 32, 33, 39, 42, 44, 45, 49, 75, 77, 79, 81, 83, 86, 88, 94, 98, 100, 102, 104, 106, 114, 118, 119, 123, 130, 131, 133, 136, 137, 138, 140, 141, 146, 147, 151, 166, 180, 183, 186, 192, 194, 198, 200, 208
adolescence, vii, ix, 29, 51, 52, 99
adolescents, xii, 46, 60, 85, 187, 202, 213, 217, 218, 219
adults, x, 44, 46, 60, 69, 78, 81, 82, 83, 84, 85, 87, 89, 90, 92, 98, 99, 100, 102, 104, 105, 106, 135, 169, 180, 187
adverse effects, viii, 2, 3, 31, 47, 87, 103, 140, 150, 176, 194, 199
adverse event, 88, 154
age, vii, ix, xi, xii, 29, 39, 40, 43, 44, 45, 46, 48, 50, 51, 52, 54, 55, 56, 60, 63, 64, 77, 78, 79, 83, 84, 86, 87, 89, 98, 99, 101, 102, 104, 106, 135, 141, 149, 154, 155, 156, 157, 159, 165, 166, 169, 177, 178, 192, 193, 195, 197, 203, 204, 205, 207, 209, 213, 214, 216
aging, viii, 23, 25, 29, 153
AIDS, 53, 67, 69, 73, 106
albumin, 44, 49, 82, 103, 104, 108, 110, 145, 164, 171, 185
alcohol abuse, 214
alcohol consumption, 218
amino acid, 94, 96, 164, 172
aminoglycosides, 21, 99, 100, 105, 142, 149, 169, 180
analgesics, xii, 94, 204, 206, 207, 208, 209, 216

anatomy, 45, 162, 164
anemia, 129, 159
anencephaly, 61, 62
antibiotic, x, 110, 113, 114, 115, 118, 119, 120, 122, 124, 179, 180, 202
antibody, 144
anticonvulsant, 104, 110
antidepressants, 20, 110, 140, 216
antiepileptic drugs, 110, 154
antiepileptics, xii, 204, 207, 209, 216
anxiolytic, 206, 208
atrophy, 67, 158, 160, 162, 164
autoimmune disease, 82, 90

B

bacteria, 53, 54, 80, 81, 102, 115, 180
bacterial conjunctivitis, 68
barbiturates, 94, 99, 174
basal metabolic rate, 87
bile, 40, 81, 101, 108
bilirubin, 103, 104, 141, 171, 179
bioavailability, 20, 29, 102, 103, 106, 135, 139, 146, 174, 186
biological fluids, 3, 27, 30, 36
biological samples, vii
biotransformation, 5, 8, 33, 36, 39, 42, 45, 76, 77, 84, 98, 123, 137, 167, 168, 169, 170, 179, 182, 183, 186
birth, vii, ix, x, 41, 43, 44, 51, 60, 61, 63, 71, 78, 79, 80, 82, 91, 92, 100, 105, 106, 109, 110, 159, 190, 197
birth weight, 105, 110
blood, 5, 6, 8, 9, 10, 12, 13, 17, 18, 33, 34, 40, 41, 44, 54, 55, 57, 76, 77, 79, 81, 85, 94, 99, 100, 104, 106, 108, 110, 119, 137, 141, 142, 143, 153, 165, 168, 170, 171, 172, 174, 177, 181
blood circulation, 76
blood flow, 8, 9, 10, 18, 40, 44, 57, 79, 81, 94, 99, 100, 137, 170, 171, 174, 182
blood pressure, 181
body clearance, 10, 37, 38, 104, 115, 122, 179
body composition, vii, 29, 82, 98, 160
body fat, 82, 99
body fluid, 5, 27, 143
body weight, ix, 20, 25, 26, 44, 77, 81, 83, 87, 98, 99, 105, 128, 129, 130, 135
bone, 158, 185
bone mass, 185
bowel, 43, 101
brain, 61, 62, 64, 67
breast feeding, 69, 103, 110
breast milk, 103

C

caffeine, 84, 186
carbamazepine, 110, 204, 207, 216
catabolism, 160, 164
central nervous system, 58, 67
chemical, 56, 80, 81, 82, 108, 157, 160, 162, 164, 168, 171, 172, 173
child mortality, 71
childcare, viii
childhood, ix, xi, 29, 51, 52, 54, 55, 61, 66, 70, 106, 153, 154, 155, 184, 185, 202
children, iii, v, vi, vii, ix, x, xi, xii, 26, 43, 44, 45, 46, 47, 49, 50, 52, 53, 54, 55, 63, 64, 65, 67, 68, 69, 70, 75, 76, 77, 78, 81, 82, 84, 85, 86, 87, 88, 90, 92, 98, 99, 102, 105, 106, 109, 110, 129, 133, 135, 150, 155, 156, 165, 166, 168, 169, 176, 177, 178, 179, 180, 181, 182, 183, 184, 185, 187, 190, 200, 202, 204, 205, 206, 207, 208, 209, 210, 211, 213, 214, 215, 216, 217, 219
children and adolescents, xii, 187, 213, 219
chloramphenicol, 86, 90, 102, 104, 130, 169, 179, 180, 182, 187
chronic renal failure, 129

circadian rhythm, 29, 106
circulation, 18, 41, 43, 78, 93, 95, 100, 106
clearance, iv, 8, 9, 10, 19, 38, 40, 84, 99, 100, 105, 119, 122, 130, 147, 168, 170, 174, 176, 178, 182, 186, 187
clinic, 2, 27, 54, 60, 73, 218
clinical application, viii, 2, 42, 137
clinical diagnosis, 136, 208
clinical trials, 31
closure, 58, 61, 62
compartments, 17, 18, 27, 30, 35, 38, 44, 83, 114, 125, 135, 167, 177
complications, 55, 63, 65, 67, 68, 98
compounds, x, 39, 40, 42, 44, 45, 81, 82, 92, 93, 94, 97, 101, 103, 142, 143, 168, 171, 187, 209
concentration, x, xi, 3, 6, 7, 8, 9, 10, 12, 13, 15, 16, 19, 20, 21, 27, 30, 32, 33, 34, 36, 37, 38, 41, 42, 44, 79, 81, 82, 83, 85, 86, 87, 93, 94, 95, 103, 104, 105, 113, 117, 118, 119, 120, 121, 122, 127, 128, 129, 131, 134, 136, 137, 139, 140, 145, 146, 148, 152, 153, 164, 166
congenital, 53, 56, 57, 58, 59, 60, 63, 71
congenital abnormalities, 56, 58
congenital heart disease, 57, 58, 59, 60, 63, 71
congestive heart failure, 206
consumption, 150, 195, 196, 202
coronary artery disease, 145
cost, 69, 149, 150, 151
cough, 54, 65, 67
creatinine, 94, 141, 192, 193
cross-sectional study, 184, 201
cyclosporine, 49, 110, 153
cytochrome, 42, 48, 83, 84, 105, 132, 165, 166, 168, 169, 170, 172, 174, 175, 177, 178, 185, 186, 187
cytochrome p450, 42, 48, 165, 166, 168, 169, 170, 172, 185, 186
cytochromes, 48, 177, 187

D

deaths, 53, 63, 64, 66, 156
decay, 32, 34, 35, 36, 116, 125
defects, 56, 57, 58, 59, 61, 71
deficiency, 46, 56, 156, 157, 160, 167, 175, 180, 184
delivery, x, 69, 73, 91, 92, 93, 98, 101, 118, 171
depression, 184, 193, 215
design, 19, 27, 32, 37, 50, 116, 120, 123, 128, 129, 152
detection, xi, 27, 69, 144, 189, 190, 191, 192, 195
developing countries, xi, 55, 64, 71, 72, 155
development, v, ix, x, 25, 27, 29, 31, 39, 47, 51, 52, 53, 56, 58, 82, 87, 92, 96, 98, 99, 111, 142, 152, 157, 158, 159, 165, 184, 199, 200, 209, 219
diarrhea, 53, 55, 65, 67, 68, 71, 193
diet, xi, 29, 43, 56, 79, 96, 101, 156, 157, 164, 165, 166, 173, 174, 183, 185, 186
dietary habits, 202
differential diagnosis, 56
diffusion, 13, 43, 78, 80, 81, 93, 95
disability, 56, 64, 215
diseases, v, ix, xi, 2, 39, 51, 52, 53, 54, 56, 57, 59, 60, 66, 72, 80, 82, 115, 131, 135, 149, 162, 167, 170, 173, 180, 190, 200, 202, 205, 206, 210
disorder, 62, 145, 215
distribution, vii, ix, xi, 5, 6, 10, 18, 23, 26, 27, 29, 31, 34, 35, 36, 37, 38, 40, 41, 44, 45, 70, 75, 76, 77, 78, 82, 83, 85, 98, 99, 100, 104, 105, 108, 115, 118, 125, 126, 129, 135, 136, 137, 147, 156, 160, 164, 167, 168, 169, 177, 181, 207
dizziness, 193
doctors, viii, 152

dosage, 21, 23, 38, 85, 87, 114, 115, 121, 130, 134, 135, 136, 138, 146, 147, 148, 152, 153, 200, 205
dosage regimen, 21, 23, 38, 115, 121, 136, 138, 147, 148, 152
dose adjustment, viii, xi, 19, 100, 134, 145, 146, 148, 149
dose-response relationship, 137, 140, 175
dosification, 87
dosing, xii, 12, 13, 19, 20, 21, 27, 32, 48, 50, 136, 150, 153, 177, 179, 204
dosing interval, 12, 13, 20, 21, 136
Down syndrome, 58, 72
drug concentrations, 6, 8, 17, 30, 31, 32, 33, 122, 138, 139, 172
drug consumption, xii, 190, 195, 196, 197, 198, 200, 202
drug delivery, 171
drug interaction, 29, 31, 132, 135, 139, 146, 170, 172, 194, 200
drug metabolism, 42, 46, 49, 50, 101, 103, 105, 166, 168, 173, 174, 178, 186
drug monitoring, vii, 3, 29, 100, 137, 141, 144, 147, 151, 152
drug reactions, 151, 186, 190, 201
drug release, 77
drug resistance, 199
drug safety, 151
drug therapy, 29, 89, 107, 131, 135, 167
drug toxicity, 167
dysentery, 52, 55, 56, 179

E

elimination, ix, 5, 6, 7, 8, 9, 10, 11, 12, 13, 17, 18, 19, 26, 27, 30, 31, 32, 33, 34, 35, 36, 37, 45, 46, 69, 76, 77, 81, 83, 85, 86, 90, 105, 114, 115, 116, 118, 119, 120, 125, 127, 130, 136, 139, 140, 141, 142, 147, 148, 150, 164, 168, 169, 170, 176, 177, 178, 181, 182
energy, 157, 160, 175, 185
environment, 92, 98, 151, 199
environmental change, 36
environmental conditions, 37
environmental factors, 45, 53, 173
enzymatic activity, 42, 169
enzyme, 8, 41, 49, 59, 144, 153, 166, 168, 170, 171, 172, 174, 175, 178, 179, 180, 182
enzyme immunoassay, 153
enzyme inhibitors, 59
enzyme-linked immunosorbent assay, 144
epilepsy, 110, 153, 206
epileptic patients, 134
equilibrium, 17, 41, 86, 97, 119, 122, 136, 142, 159, 160, 181
excretion, ix, 5, 27, 29, 31, 36, 39, 40, 42, 45, 46, 75, 76, 77, 78, 85, 86, 98, 105, 106, 135, 137, 168, 169, 176, 183, 185
external environment, 43, 78
extraction, 9, 10, 143, 144, 171

F

falls, 43, 64
families, 68, 172, 196, 214
fat, 41, 44, 45, 83, 99, 160, 163
fatty acids, 82, 97
fetal circulation, 41, 93, 95
fetal compartments, 97
fetal death, 92
fetal development, 82
fetal growth, 41, 96
fetus, v, x, 39, 40, 41, 42, 49, 50, 56, 83, 91, 92, 93, 95, 97, 99, 108, 111
fever, 54, 65, 67, 193
fluid, 41, 61, 98, 142, 163
food, 62, 79, 80, 101, 114, 156, 157, 184, 186, 196
food intake, 156, 186
formula, 38, 79, 122, 130, 196

G

gastric lavage, 208
gastrointestinal, xi, 40, 43, 48, 49, 64, 78, 79, 89, 100, 101, 174, 179, 190, 194, 199, 200
gastrointestinal tract, 43, 78, 179
gentamicin, viii, 2, 105, 134, 150, 153, 180, 181, 183, 187
gestation, 57, 60, 93, 98, 105, 197
gestational age, 45, 46, 86, 100, 110, 141
gestational period, 92
glucose, 94, 95, 175, 185
growth, v, 25, 28, 29, 31, 39, 41, 47, 55, 69, 87, 92, 93, 96, 97, 98, 106, 157, 158, 159, 165, 184, 209
growth factor, 96
guidelines, 109, 131, 201, 202

H

haemophilus influenzae, 54, 70
half-life, 6, 11, 12, 13, 17, 18, 19, 32, 35, 45, 46, 83, 84, 85, 90, 105, 115, 119, 130, 136, 141, 142, 147, 176, 178, 181, 182
headache, 65, 193
health, viii, ix, x, xii, 26, 51, 52, 54, 64, 72, 91, 151, 152, 156, 190, 191, 196, 199, 213, 216, 217, 218
health problems, 190
heart diseases, 57, 58, 59, 60, 63
heart failure, 59, 100, 181
heart rate, 141, 192, 193
height, 28, 77, 87, 141, 177, 192, 193, 197, 198
hemodialysis, 132, 185
hepatocytes, 178, 179
hepatomegaly, 59, 60
Hirschsprung, 58
history, 56, 87, 215, 218
HIV, 53, 67, 68, 69, 70, 73
homeostasis, 158, 159, 162
hormones, 82, 96, 98
hospitalization, xii, 103, 204, 205, 209
human, 2, 29, 31, 42, 48, 49, 65, 68, 79, 90, 93, 96, 98, 107, 108, 109, 149, 167, 178, 187
human immunodeficiency virus, 68
human milk, 79
hypersensitivity, 78, 191, 194

I

immaturity, viii, 25, 29, 47, 84, 85, 87, 98, 106, 214
immune response, 67
immunization, 53, 54, 68
immunosuppression, 69
impregnation, 141
impulsiveness, 215
in utero, 61, 110
in vitro, 166, 169, 187
in vivo, 95, 168, 171, 172, 174
incubation period, 65
individual variability, viii, 1, 2, 137, 138, 148, 149, 170
individualization, 31, 123, 135
infancy, 55, 71
infants, ix, xii, 29, 43, 44, 45, 46, 50, 51, 52, 59, 60, 69, 70, 78, 81, 83, 86, 89, 90, 101, 105, 110, 165, 202, 204, 209
infection, x, 53, 54, 64, 65, 66, 67, 68, 113, 115, 123, 149, 185
ingestion, xii, 203, 204, 208, 209, 218, 219
injury, iv, 72, 205, 214
insulin, 40, 85, 96
insulin-like growth factor, 96
intellectual disabilities, 58
intensive care unit, 150, 153
intoxication, 47, 87, 143, 169, 195, 210
intrauterine, x, 41, 56, 58, 91, 92

intravenously, 33, 117, 122, 180
ionization, 40, 79, 82, 86, 94
iron, 94, 96
iron supplement, 96
iron transport, 96
issues, ix, xi, 51, 52, 189, 196

K

kidney, 8, 41, 42, 85, 167, 169, 179 181, 182, 186
kinetic, 5, 6, 30, 33, 35, 36, 37, 38, 41, 47, 48, 50, 87, 116, 117, 119, 140, 146, 169
kinetic model, 116, 117
kinetic parameters, 37, 38

L

laboratory tests, 190, 205
LADME, v, ix, 75, 76, 77, 109
life expectancy, 63
lifetime, 7
liver, 8, 42, 49, 65, 83, 98, 103, 105, 165, 167, 168, 170, 171, 172, 174, 175, 176, 186, 187
liver cirrhosis, 171
liver disease, 103, 186
liver enzymes, 49, 168, 171
liver function tests, 170, 171
loading dose, 6, 13, 21, 122, 128, 129
local anesthetic, 94, 95

M

macronutrients, 174
maintenance dose, 19, 20, 122, 129, 130, 131, 141
malaria, 53, 64, 65, 66, 72, 73
malnourished children, 166, 168, 176, 178, 179, 185, 187
malnourishment, 156
malnutrition, xi, 47, 55, 90, 96, 155, 156, 157, 158, 159, 160, 161, 162, 163, 164, 165, 166, 167, 168, 169, 170, 175, 176, 177, 179, 180, 181, 183, 184, 185, 188, 196
mammalian cells, 186
maturity, viii, 25, 29, 40, 46, 81, 86
measles, 53, 66, 67, 68, 73
medical, vii, ix, x, 2, 25, 31, 38, 121, 133, 141, 144, 150, 152, 162, 181, 184, 194, 195, 205
medical care, vii
medication, xii, 2, 32, 54, 103, 107, 110, 192, 193, 197, 198, 201, 202, 204, 209, 216
medicine, viii, ix, 1, 25, 31, 32, 35, 36, 37, 39, 40, 41, 121, 136, 137, 209
mellitus, 56
membranes, 77, 93, 94, 96
meningitis, 54, 179
mental health, 214, 218
mesenchymal stem cells, 109
metabolic alkalosis, 141
metabolic change, 157, 166
metabolic pathways, 42, 45, 169, 170
metabolism, ix, 23, 29, 31, 42, 45, 46, 49, 50, 69, 75, 76, 78, 80, 83, 84, 85, 97, 98, 101, 103, 105, 106, 108, 109, 146, 154, 157, 159, 166, 168, 169, 171, 172, 173, 174, 175, 176, 178, 185, 186, 187
metabolites, 5, 30, 43, 45, 76, 77, 84, 90, 139, 146, 169, 170, 172, 176, 179
metabolized, 46, 77, 85, 172, 175, 176
metabolizing, 41, 42, 45, 49, 169, 170, 179, 209
methods of suicide, 216
metronidazole, 123, 124, 168, 177, 178, 179, 182, 187
Mexico, 1, 25, 51, 71, 75, 113, 133, 149, 155, 156, 183, 189, 190, 200, 202, 203, 205, 209, 213, 218, 219

micronutrients, 183
microorganism, 118, 122, 174
microsomal oxidation, 176
microsomes, 166, 174, 178, 187
minimum concentration, 3, 131, 136, 179
mortality, xi, 52, 55, 56, 63, 64, 66, 67, 68, 70, 150, 155, 156
mortality rate, xi, 64, 155, 156

N

neonates, 50, 89, 90, 98, 100, 101, 102, 103, 104, 105, 110, 178, 187
neural tube defects, 56, 58, 71
newborn, v, ix, x, 29, 40, 42, 43, 44, 45, 46, 49, 50, 51, 52, 69, 70, 78, 80, 81, 82, 83, 84, 86, 87, 91, 92, 93, 98, 99, 101, 102, 103, 104, 107, 108, 109, 111, 143, 180, 201
non-steroidal anti-inflammatory drugs, 111
nutrients, x, 91, 94, 101, 156, 157, 162
nutrition, vi, 53, 68, 155, 157, 160, 176, 182, 183, 184, 185, 186
nutritional deficiencies, xi, 155, 173
nutritional status, ix, 25, 29, 68, 145, 173, 174, 183, 185

O

old age, 29
organism, ix, 3, 5, 10, 18, 25, 26, 30, 31, 32, 33, 39, 40, 41, 42, 43, 46, 76, 81, 87, 116, 117, 119, 135, 136, 156, 158, 160, 162, 164, 167
organs, 5, 8, 9, 10, 18, 28, 32, 69, 77, 92, 98, 99, 114, 162
overweight, 56, 184
oxidation, 45, 46, 85, 168, 175, 176, 187

P

pain, 65, 193, 218
palpitations, 193
parents, 69, 196, 214, 215, 217
pathogens, 66, 149
pathology, 55, 160, 162, 164, 194
pathophysiological, 38, 47, 104, 160, 166
pathophysiology, 57, 165
pathway, ix, 45, 75, 76, 169, 181, 182
pediatric, vi, vii, ix, x, xi, xii, 29, 48, 50, 51, 52, 53, 69, 70, 73, 88, 89, 113, 135, 143, 145, 149, 153, 156, 157, 169, 170, 179, 183, 189, 190, 192, 201, 202, 203, 204, 205, 206, 208, 209, 213, 219
pediatric infectology, x, 113
pediatrician, x, 133
penicillin, 46, 54, 78, 86, 181
perfusion, 49, 59, 100, 168
perinatal, ix, 51, 52, 53, 56
pH, 40, 43, 78, 79, 80, 86, 100, 106, 174
phagocytosis, x, 54, 92, 113
pharmaceutical, x, 38, 75, 76, 141, 151
pharmacodynamic, x, 92, 115, 131
pharmacoepidemiology, vi, xi, 189, 190, 195, 198
pharmacokinetic, v, viii, x, 1, 2, 3, 5, 18, 19, 22, 23, 25, 26, 27, 29, 30, 31, 32, 36, 37, 38, 39, 48, 69, 76, 78, 82, 89, 90, 92, 98, 113, 115, 116, 118, 119, 122, 123, 128, 129, 131, 135, 139, 141, 147, 148, 152, 153, 154, 166, 167, 168, 169, 170, 172, 176, 177, 178,180, 182, 187, 196, 204
pharmacokinetic parameters, 19, 27, 31, 36, 37, 69, 115, 116, 119, 123, 128, 129, 139, 147, 148, 177, 178
pharmacological, ix, xi, 2, 3, 23, 26, 30, 39, 47, 77, 85, 87, 88, 89, 98, 106, 109, 121, 133, 135, 136, 137, 147, 151, 167, 191, 201, 208

pharmacological response, 26, 30, 136, 147, 167
pharmacological success, ix, 26
pharmacology, 27, 30, 50, 76, 88, 186, 191, 193, 194
pharmacotherapy, 69, 101
pharmacovigilance, vi, xi, 150, 151, 152, 154, 189, 190, 191, 201
phenotype, 132
phenytoin, 83, 89, 90, 95, 104, 134, 137, 142, 145, 146, 152, 153, 154, 204, 207
physicians, viii, 1, 2, 20, 26, 27, 47, 135, 148, 151, 152, 154, 199, 216, 217
physicochemical characteristics, 94
physicochemical properties, x, 81, 91, 94
physiological factors, 87, 209
physiology, 27, 48, 50, 89, 164
physiopathology, 77
placenta, x, 39, 40, 41, 42, 91, 92, 93, 94, 95, 96, 97, 107, 108, 109
placental barrier, 108
plasma concentration, viii, ix, xii, 2, 3, 5, 6, 8, 15, 26, 27, 33, 34, 36, 38, 89, 90, 116, 117, 118, 120, 124, 125, 128, 129, 131, 135, 136, 152, 171, 180, 203, 204, 206, 207, 208
plasma levels, viii, ix, 3, 26, 96, 137, 154, 164, 180
plasma proteins, 40, 42, 44, 46, 49, 82, 83, 95, 104, 110, 145, 181
pneumonia, 52, 53, 54, 55, 67, 68, 70, 149
poisoning, xii, 64, 203, 204, 205, 206, 207, 208, 209, 210, 216
population, vii, xi, xii, 52, 63, 68, 69, 71, 88, 106, 135, 149, 152, 153, 155, 156, 169, 191, 192, 195, 196, 203, 204, 206, 207, 208, 209, 214, 219
pregnancy, 40, 41, 42, 48, 56, 62, 63, 69, 93, 96, 107, 108, 109, 110, 111
premature infant, 45, 101
preschool, ix, 29, 51, 52, 159
prescription, xi, 26, 39, 98, 152, 189, 190, 191, 195, 199, 202
preterm infants, 44, 45, 46, 60
prevention, 52, 53, 62, 64, 66, 68, 70, 72, 73, 89, 139, 149, 185, 214, 216, 217
prognosis, 63, 159, 172
protein binding, 40, 44, 48, 82, 90, 95, 100, 103, 104, 137, 139, 145, 146, 175, 188
protein deficit, 157
proteins, 42, 44, 77, 79, 81, 82, 83, 95, 103, 104, 141, 145, 157, 160, 164, 165, 166, 168, 171, 172, 175, 181
psychiatric disease, 215
psychiatric disorder, 214, 215, 219
psychiatric illness, xii, 213, 215
psychotropic drugs, 3
public health, xi, 155, 214

Q

QT interval, 210
qualitative differences, 44
quality of life, 63
quantification, xi, 27, 29, 37, 134, 142, 143, 144, 170, 171

R

rash, 193
receptor, 3, 4, 98, 145, 167, 168, 210
receptor sites, 98
recovery, 177, 180, 181, 182, 183, 187
renal dysfunction, 130
renal excretion, 39, 40, 46, 77, 85, 86, 106, 169, 180, 183
renal failure, 103, 129, 130, 167
resources, 26, 151, 195, 199
risk, x, xii, 27, 29, 47, 55, 56, 57, 62, 69, 70, 76, 86, 87, 88, 100, 102, 106, 113, 120, 131, 140, 149, 156, 169, 177, 203, 204, 214, 215, 217

rosiglitazone, 108

S

salicylates, 82, 95, 104, 196
school, ix, 29, 51, 52, 156, 202, 216
school children, 46, 85, 202
science, 5
secretion, 23, 46, 79, 86, 100, 106, 143
sedatives, 216
seizure, 123, 134, 154
self-medication, xii, 204, 209
sepsis, 90, 134
septum, 59, 60
serotonin, 215
serum, 61, 63, 99, 102, 104, 109, 134, 135, 136, 140, 142, 144, 146, 150, 153, 165, 171, 179, 192, 193
serum albumin, 104, 171
serum drug concentration, 135
sex, 29, 141, 175, 192
skin, 41, 102, 158, 159, 193
social change, ix, 51, 52
sodium, 55, 94, 110, 163
solubility, 18, 40, 45, 48, 79, 94
steady-state average concentration, 115
stenosis, 58, 59, 60
stomach, 79, 114, 193
subacute, 158, 160
substrate, 166, 170, 172
suicidal behavior, xii, 213, 214, 215, 216, 218, 219
suicidal ideation, xii, 213, 214, 215, 216
suicide, xii, 213, 214, 215, 216, 217, 218, 219
suicide attempts, 219
suicide rate, 214
surgical intervention, 190, 205
symptoms, 65, 139, 146, 156, 184, 192, 194
syndrome, 56, 61, 62, 72, 80, 86, 167
synthesis, 31, 98, 164
systolic murmur, 59, 60

T

tachycardia, 59, 60, 139
tachypnea, 54, 59
therapeutic, vi, vii, viii, ix, x, xi, 1, 2, 3, 4, 19, 20, 25, 26, 27, 29, 31, 32, 39, 47, 50, 75, 77, 85, 86, 87, 88, 89, 90, 101, 102, 114, 118, 119, 120, 121, 122, 123, 128, 129, 130, 133, 134, 135, 136, 137, 139, 140, 142, 144, 145, 146, 148, 149, 152, 153, 156, 162, 168, 169, 170, 171, 177, 181, 183, 195, 196, 204, 206, 207, 208
therapeutic agents, 135
therapeutic drug monitoring, vi, x, 50, 89, 90, 133, 134, 135, 152, 153, 171, 206, 207, 208
therapeutic effect, 101, 122, 137, 145, 149
therapeutic regimens, xi, 27, 156, 170, 183
therapeutic use, 31, 162
therapeutic window, 32, 118, 120, 121, 122
therapy, vii, 2, 19, 29, 31, 66, 89, 107, 109, 110, 115, 131, 135, 140, 150, 152, 167, 173, 181
tissue, 18, 41, 42, 46, 61, 62, 79, 83, 86, 92, 99, 100, 157, 158, 160, 164, 168
toddlers, 29
toxic, viii, ix, 2, 3, 32, 39, 54, 75, 76, 77, 80, 81, 86, 92, 100, 102, 104, 120, 137, 145, 148, 149, 175, 180, 204, 210
toxic effect, ix, 39, 75, 77, 80, 86, 100, 102, 104, 137, 175
toxic substances, 92, 103, 210
toxicity, viii, x, 3, 47, 83, 87, 101, 104, 111, 113, 120, 131, 137, 138, 139, 140, 141, 146, 147, 167, 173, 174, 181
trace elements, 166
transference, 30, 93, 94, 95, 96, 177
treatment, vii, viii, x, xii, 1, 2, 27, 31, 32, 37, 53, 54, 59, 60, 61, 65, 68, 69, 70, 73,

88, 89, 100, 105, 110, 114, 115, 116, 118, 119, 120, 121, 122, 123, 128, 129, 130, 132, 133, 134, 135, 140, 141, 147, 149, 152, 154, 167, 169, 180, 191, 195, 200, 202, 203, 205, 206, 208, 210, 218
treatment regimen, vii, 31, 32, 37, 105, 114, 115, 116, 118, 119, 120, 121, 122, 123, 128, 129, 130, 167

U

ultrasound, 63
undernutrition, 169
unintentional drug poisoning, vi, xii, 203, 205, 206, 209
urinary retention, 193
urinary tract infection, 56
urine, 40, 42, 86, 143, 172, 176, 179, 181
usual dose, 130, 191

V

vaccination, 52, 54, 68
vaccine, 54, 66, 68, 73
vancomycin, 100, 187
vascular system, 18, 39, 77
viruses, 66
vitamin A, 56, 68, 184
vitamin D, 184, 185
vitamin K, 108
volume of distribution, 10, 17, 18, 23, 37, 38, 41, 82, 115, 129, 147, 177, 181
vomiting, 65, 68, 100, 101, 103, 193

W

weight, ix, 20, 25, 26, 39, 44, 77, 81, 83, 87, 94, 98, 99, 100, 102, 105, 109, 110, 123, 128, 129, 130, 135, 141, 156, 158, 159, 160, 162, 164, 175, 177, 192, 193, 197, 198, 199
worldwide, 53, 54, 55, 56, 66, 88, 214

Y

young adults, 178

Z

zero-order, 5, 8, 13